"With the topic of gender identity becoming very high p[rofile in e]... [re]sour[ces] of theatre techniques to address this subject are few [a]nd [for between]... [manual embeds] practical exploration of gender themes into those accessible, heuristic and relevant activities which vitalise the learning journey of a theatre student. This publication is an essential resource for every school, college or university department as a seminal handbook in the contemporary studies of theatre and gender."

Michał J. Pasternak *FRSA FCCT, Examining Board Representative for IB DP group 6 the Arts. HLM International Schools Theatre Association [ISTA]*

"In our rapidly changing and complex world, educators have a responsibility to place issues of diversity, equity and inclusion at the heart of their teaching. In order to authentically and meaningfully do so, we must educate ourselves, critically examine our practice and acquire the skills and tools required. What better way to do this than by learning from an experienced international theatre educator who models exemplary practice in the theatre classroom. Grounded in research, covering the full breadth of a theatre curriculum and brimming with practical exercises and activities, *Teaching Drama With, Without and About Gender* is both a must and a gift for all international theatre teachers."

Sally Robertson, *Executive Director, International Schools Theatre Association*

"A very practical guide for using drama as a learning process for questioning, re-imagining and re-affirming the complexities of identity. This book provides an essential toolkit and rationale for practising drama as the art form of being human in all its variety. Students will benefit from the openness of the learning approach and the opportunities through drama to safely challenge gendered pre-conceptions of identity and to imagine themselves differently."

Jonothan Neelands *PhD, DSc, FRSA., Academic Director for Cultural Partnerships, University of Warwick*

Teaching Drama With, Without and About Gender

This exciting new book offers practical resources and lesson plans for exploring gender in the drama curriculum. It looks at how theatre performances throughout history have played with the concept of identity and gender and explains why drama lessons can provide a safe and considerate space for thinking about gender.

Drawing on theatre history, world theatre, theatre forms and theatre theory, each chapter focuses on key topics that will challenge students to play and explore gender roles as they choose. Introducing a new drama vocabulary drawn from archaeology and cartography, this book includes a wide range of materials for excavation from traditional stories, contemporary children's literature, Greek mythology, Elizabethan and Restoration theatre, Japanese and Chinese theatre, mask, and physical theatre.

Providing new insight into how existing drama units can be redefined to create a space where the exploration of gender identity is not only allowed but something exciting and joyful to focus on, this is an essential resource for all drama teachers.

Jo Riley, a graduate of Cambridge University, learnt Mandarin to study at the Central Academy of Drama in Beijing. With over 20 years' international experience she has led workshops, published, translated and edited extensively on Chinese theatre, European theatre history and intercultural theatre. Her special focus is the kinetic language of bodies in space, and bodies as pictograms of an idea.

Teaching Drama With, Without and About Gender

Resources, Ideas and Lesson Plans for Students 11–18

Jo Riley

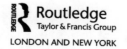
Routledge
Taylor & Francis Group

LONDON AND NEW YORK

Cover image: © Getty Images

First published 2022
by Routledge
2 Park Square, Milton Park, Abingdon, Oxon OX14 4RN

and by Routledge
605 Third Avenue, New York, NY 10158

Routledge is an imprint of the Taylor & Francis Group, an informa business

British Library Cataloguing-in-Publication Data
A catalogue record for this book is available from the British Library

Library of Congress Cataloging-in-Publication Data
Names: Riley, Jo, author.
Title: Teaching drama with, without and about gender: resources, ideas and lesson plans for students 11–18 / Jo Riley.
Description: Abingdon, Oxon; New York: Routledge, 2022 |
Includes bibliographical references and index.
Identifiers: LCCN 2021025440 | ISBN 9780367531768 (hardback) |
ISBN 9780367531812 (paperback) | ISBN 9781003080800 (ebook)
Subjects: LCSH: Drama—Study and teaching (Secondary). | Gender identity in the theater. | Gender identity in literature.
Classification: LCC PN1701 .R55 2022 | DDC 792.0712—dc23
LC record available at https://lccn.loc.gov/2021025440

ISBN: 978-0-367-53176-8 (hbk)
ISBN: 978-0-367-53181-2 (pbk)
ISBN: 978-1-003-08080-0 (ebk)

DOI: 10.4324/9781003080800

Typeset in Helvetica
by codeMantra

For Michael, Lucia, Dylan and Aminta

CONTENTS

CHAPTER 2
About gender - seeking identity

CHAPTER 3
Without gender - mask

CHAPTER 5
With gender – world theatre

TABLES

FIGURES

ACKNOWLEDGEMENTS

I am deeply grateful to Phillippa Lior for the beautiful drawings of facial expressions as mask templates; to Teresa Riley for extensive and detailed editing; to Eni Xu for help in formatting images; and drama friends and colleagues for their kind and wise ideas and revisions.

Resources

All the terms in the list below come from a variety of sources, but principally:

Barker, Meg-John and Julia Scheele. *Queer. A Graphic History*. London: Icon Books, 2016.

Chappell, Sharon Verner, Karyl E. Ketchum, and Lisa Richardson. *Gender Diversity and LGBTQ Inclusion in K-12 Schools*. New York and London: Routledge, 2018.

GLSEN. *The Safe Space Kit*. New York: GLSEN, 2016.

Mardell, Ashley. *The ABC's of LGBT+*. Mango Media, 2016.

Storck, Kelly. *The Gender Identity Workbook for Kids*. New Harbinger, 2018.

Kuklin, Susan. *Beyond Magenta. Transgender Teens Speak Out*. Somerville, MA: Candlewick Press, 2014.

GLOSSARY

Ally

A member of the majority or dominant group who works to end oppression by recognizing their own privilege and supporting or advocating for the oppressed population.

Camp

Camp can consist of parody, exaggeration, theatricality, irony and humour. Camp performances can parody gender and sexuality. Camp is not synonymous with gay.

Cisgender or Cis

When a person is cisgender or cis, this means they identify exclusively with the gender/sex they were assigned at birth (e.g. my friend Emily was assigned female at birth and identifies as a woman. She is a cis-gendered woman).

FTM

Female to male, a person assigned female at birth but who identifies as male.

Gay

A person who is emotionally and/or physically attracted to some members of the same gender. Gay often refers to a male-identified person who is emotionally and/or physically attracted to some other males. It is also used as a derogatory term to describe a thing, a person or a behaviour that does not meet the approval of the group.

Gender

The socially constructed roles, behaviours, activities and attributes that a given society considers appropriate for men and women. Gender varies between cultures and over time. There is a broad variation in the ways in which individuals experience and express gender.

In the context of individual self, gender is the state of being a man, a woman, both, neither, somewhere in between or something entirely different. In the context of society, gender is a system of classification rooted in social ideas about masculinity and femininity. Gender is what you do, not who you are.

Gender binary

The idea that there are only two genders – male and female.

Gender expression

The many ways in which a person chooses to communicate gender to themselves and others, or, in other words, the demonstration of one's gender. It describes how someone expresses their gender to the world (clothing, dress, mannerisms, speech, etc.).

Gender fluid

This term describes someone whose gender may change or who feels like a mix of genders.

Gender identity

How an individual identifies in terms of their gender, or how someone feels on the inside. Gender identity reflects a deeply felt sense of being a female, male, somewhere in between or not within these categories.

LGBTQ+ or LGBTQIA

Lesbian, Gay, Bisexual, Transgender, Q can represent questioning or queer, I stands for intersex, and A for Ally or Asexual. Sometimes the latter terms are all combined together as + which also includes any other identities that are not straight and/or cisgender. It's an umbrella term that refers to identities that do not conform to dominant societal norms.

Man

Someone who identifies as a man.

MTF

Male to female, someone who was assigned male at birth but who identifies as female.

Non-binary

A person who may have a gender that is both male and female or neither male or female something else completely. It describes someone who feels they do not belong to the eith system of either male or female.

Pronouns

She, her, hers, herself
He, him, his, himself
They, them, theirs, themselves
Ze, hir/Zir, Hirs/Zirs/Hirself (Zirself)

Queer

A term used to describe a sexual orientation, gender identity or gender expression that does not conform to societal norms. Used as a neutral or positive term now, although in the past it was a term of extreme abuse. Queer is a term used to describe any identity that is not cisgender and/or not heterosexual. It has had many different meanings in different times and places. It originally referred to strangeness or difference.

Queer theory

Is all about breaking down opposing binary systems (male/female) which suggest that people in the world are either this or that. Queer theory is based on the idea of a fluid gender identity. In the late 1800s, 'queer' was an abusive term for people attracted to the same sex. Queer has also been used as a more general term of abuse in the same way that 'gay' is used to imply something is not nice or good.

Transgender

Someone whose gender is different from their sex/gender assigned at birth. Sometimes this identity is associated with having undergone and/or wanting to undergo some kind of medical transition. The term describes a wide range of identities, expressions and experiences. Includes those whose gender assigned at birth does not match their internal sense of gender id. Not all gender-nonconforming individuals consider themselves transgender.

Transgender man

meone who was assigned female at birth and who identifies as male.

sgender woman

one who was assigned male at birth and who identifies as female.

on

ss of accepting oneself and/or pursuing changes in order to affirm a particular gender ve feelings of being 'in the wrong body' or body dysphoria.

identifies as a woman.

You are what you say you are.

Introduction

The learner-teacher-learner

My first contact with drama teachers was reading Keith Johnstone. I was immediately struck by the personal stories in the book. He revealed that school made him 'crippled and unfit for life' (Johnstone 10), and he comments on his poor success, since he felt that education was having a negative effect on his well-being. As a young adult, he reconnected with his childhood-self and encourages his reader to do the same to rediscover that child-like fearless curiosity and impulse that liberates creative endeavour. It is a thoroughly exposing opening to a book about teaching drama – but it impressed me because it placed Johnstone on an equal footing with his students and readers. The teacher was claiming to be a student, still learning, and Johnstone quotes his own teacher citing Daoist philosophy, 'To know yet to think one does not know is best.... The sage does not hoard. Having bestowed all he has on others, he is richer still . . . the way of the sage is bountiful and does not contend' (Johnstone 20).

The aim of this book is definitely not to teach anyone about anything. I must leap to admit my debt to colleagues and artists around the world from whom I have learned and am still learning. This is not a prescriptive 'how to' book or a book that will radically change your already outstanding practice in the drama classroom. I'm hoping it might simply be a pebble in your shoe as you walk the drama curriculum, reminding you that once in a while, it is important for the well-being of all the students in the class to raise the question of gender and identity explicitly. The ideas in the book draw from the regular drama curriculum – there is nothing difficult, new or complex to understand that you don't already know. But the lens on the curriculum is different, drawing deliberately and explicitly on issues with, without and about gender that might easily be accommodated into your present teaching.

Following Johnstone's model, and my Chinese masters at the Central Academy of Beijing where I learned as an apprentice, following my master's every move (there were no texts or theoretical treatises or even handbooks – everything was transmitted by process of imitation), I have also started every chapter of this book with a personal story – reluctantly, because I am not naturally expansive about my life, but because I hope to show you that I am on the same journey

DOI: 10.4324/9781003080800-1

as you and perhaps your students, trying to understand a gendered perspective in the drama classroom and feeling my way as I go.

Everyone in the drama ensemble has a story to share, and every story is valuable and valued.

My first story

Here is my first story, the story that led me to thinking about changing the way I teach drama.

This unit was taught by my mentor, Jerry Strachan. I had arrived in the classroom with little classroom teaching experience, and, instead of talking me through the steps of it, showing me guiding questions, concepts, criteria, rubrics and skills to be learnt, Jerry simply took me into the studio and said, 'watch me'. Week for week, I followed how he taught, joining in with him in Teacher-in-Role and warm-up games where there were no clear divisions in the entire ensemble between who was learning and who was teaching. Following his example, I set the students to devise monologues based on a starting point, 'Perfect' by Alanis Morissette. It's about parental pressure to be perfect. A student approached me and asked if they could perform their monologue while ripping up the dress Mum insists their character wear. Can they take a dress from the costume room and rip it up on stage? Of course, no problem, great idea, go for it. But the idea slid into the undergrowth and was never mentioned again. The disappearance of a great idea came about because the environment I had created for the ensemble was not yet, and by no means, providing a space where all great ideas are worth a shot, an exploration, a discovery, a building, a trashing and a beginning again. I thought I had been giving that, but clearly, I was wrong. It was time to find out what I could learn to do it better. I started to research gender in education.

To ostracize

This word, such a mean word, has been in the English language since the 16th century, but it draws from an ancient Greek custom of getting rid of anyone who threatened the freedom of the people or who was simply embarrassing to the state. The word actually means a piece of pottery or bone. It was on such scraps of ceramic, shell or bone that citizens could inscribe the name of anyone they wanted to eliminate from society for ten years. The shards were anonymously dropped in a jar, counted and, provided enough people participated, the citizen with the most votes was banished with no chance of appeal. The social shunning of people who don't seem to fit, who may be 'embarrassing' to the dominant peer group, is, sadly, still a part of school and classroom communities. Not belonging, being different in some way, feeling different, or not conforming to the group's decided norms is a blueprint for being shunned, picked on, picked out, harassed and bullied. According to a 2011 National School Climate Survey in the United States, schools remain 'hostile environments for a distressing number of students' (Kosciw, Palmer and Greytak 4). It was found that 84.9% students heard the term 'gay' used in a pejorative way at school; 61.4% heard negative remarks about gender expression, including some coming from teachers and other staff at school (Wilson 84). That last comment is particularly disturbing. Another study drawn from student responses showed:

63.5% of students felt unsafe because of their sexual orientation or gender identity.
81.9% of students felt unsafe because of verbal harassment.
38% of students felt unsafe because of fear of physical harassment.
18.3% of students were physically harassed.
55.2% of students suffered cyber bullying.

Queer

A term used to describe a sexual orientation, gender identity or gender expression that does not conform to societal norms. Used as a neutral or positive term now, although in the past it was a term of extreme abuse. Queer is a term used to describe any identity that is not cisgender and/or not heterosexual. It has had many different meanings in different times and places. It originally referred to strangeness or difference.

Queer theory

Is all about breaking down opposing binary systems (male/female) which suggest that people in the world are either this or that. Queer theory is based on the idea of a fluid gender identity. In the late 1800s, 'queer' was an abusive term for people attracted to the same sex. Queer has also been used as a more general term of abuse in the same way that 'gay' is used to imply something is not nice or good.

Transgender

Someone whose gender is different from their sex/gender assigned at birth. Sometimes this identity is associated with having undergone and/or wanting to undergo some kind of medical transition. The term describes a wide range of identities, expressions and experiences. Includes those whose gender assigned at birth does not match their internal sense of gender id. Not all gender-nonconforming individuals consider themselves transgender.

Transgender man

Someone who was assigned female at birth and who identifies as male.

Transgender woman

Someone who was assigned male at birth and who identifies as female.

Transition

The process of accepting oneself and/or pursuing changes in order to affirm a particular gender or resolve feelings of being 'in the wrong body' or body dysphoria.

Woman

Someone who identifies as a woman.

You are what you say you are.

In the context of individual self, gender is the state of being a man, a woman, both, neither, somewhere in between or something entirely different. In the context of society, gender is a system of classification rooted in social ideas about masculinity and femininity. Gender is what you do, not who you are.

Gender binary

The idea that there are only two genders – male and female.

Gender expression

The many ways in which a person chooses to communicate gender to themselves and others, or, in other words, the demonstration of one's gender. It describes how someone expresses their gender to the world (clothing, dress, mannerisms, speech, etc.).

Gender fluid

This term describes someone whose gender may change or who feels like a mix of genders.

Gender identity

How an individual identifies in terms of their gender, or how someone feels on the inside. Gender identity reflects a deeply felt sense of being a female, male, somewhere in between or not within these categories.

LGBTQ+ or LGBTQIA

Lesbian, Gay, Bisexual, Transgender, Q can represent questioning or queer, I stands for intersex, and A for Ally or Asexual. Sometimes the latter terms are all combined together as + which also includes any other identities that are not straight and/or cisgender. It's an umbrella term that refers to identities that do not conform to dominant societal norms.

Man

Someone who identifies as a man.

MTF

Male to female, someone who was assigned male at birth but who identifies as female.

Non-binary

A person who may have a gender that is both male and female or neither male or female or something else completely. It describes someone who feels they do not belong to the either/or system of either male or female.

Pronouns

She, her, hers, herself
He, him, his, himself
They, them, theirs, themselves
Ze, hir/Zir, Hirs/Zirs/Hirself (Zirself)

Introduction

The learner-teacher-learner

My first contact with drama teachers was reading Keith Johnstone. I was immediately struck by the personal stories in the book. He revealed that school made him 'crippled and unfit for life' (Johnstone 10), and he comments on his poor success, since he felt that education was having a negative effect on his well-being. As a young adult, he reconnected with his childhood-self and encourages his reader to do the same to rediscover that child-like fearless curiosity and impulse that liberates creative endeavour. It is a thoroughly exposing opening to a book about teaching drama – but it impressed me because it placed Johnstone on an equal footing with his students and readers. The teacher was claiming to be a student, still learning, and Johnstone quotes his own teacher citing Daoist philosophy, 'To know yet to think one does not know is best.... The sage does not hoard. Having bestowed all he has on others, he is richer still . . . the way of the sage is bountiful and does not contend' (Johnstone 20).

The aim of this book is definitely not to teach anyone about anything. I must leap to admit my debt to colleagues and artists around the world from whom I have learned and am still learning. This is not a prescriptive 'how to' book or a book that will radically change your already outstanding practice in the drama classroom. I'm hoping it might simply be a pebble in your shoe as you walk the drama curriculum, reminding you that once in a while, it is important for the well-being of all the students in the class to raise the question of gender and identity explicitly. The ideas in the book draw from the regular drama curriculum – there is nothing difficult, new or complex to understand that you don't already know. But the lens on the curriculum is different, drawing deliberately and explicitly on issues with, without and about gender that might easily be accommodated into your present teaching.

Following Johnstone's model, and my Chinese masters at the Central Academy of Beijing where I learned as an apprentice, following my master's every move (there were no texts or theoretical treatises or even handbooks – everything was transmitted by process of imitation), I have also started every chapter of this book with a personal story – reluctantly, because I am not naturally expansive about my life, but because I hope to show you that I am on the same journey

DOI: 10.4324/9781003080800-1

as you and perhaps your students, trying to understand a gendered perspective in the drama classroom and feeling my way as I go.

Everyone in the drama ensemble has a story to share, and every story is valuable and valued.

My first story

Here is my first story, the story that led me to thinking about changing the way I teach drama.

This unit was taught by my mentor, Jerry Strachan. I had arrived in the classroom with little classroom teaching experience, and, instead of talking me through the steps of it, showing me guiding questions, concepts, criteria, rubrics and skills to be learnt, Jerry simply took me into the studio and said, 'watch me'. Week for week, I followed how he taught, joining in with him in Teacher-in-Role and warm-up games where there were no clear divisions in the entire ensemble between who was learning and who was teaching. Following his example, I set the students to devise monologues based on a starting point, 'Perfect' by Alanis Morissette. It's about parental pressure to be perfect. A student approached me and asked if they could perform their monologue while ripping up the dress Mum insists their character wear. Can they take a dress from the costume room and rip it up on stage? Of course, no problem, great idea, go for it. But the idea slid into the undergrowth and was never mentioned again. The disappearance of a great idea came about because the environment I had created for the ensemble was not yet, and by no means, providing a space where all great ideas are worth a shot, an exploration, a discovery, a building, a trashing and a beginning again. I thought I had been giving that, but clearly, I was wrong. It was time to find out what I could learn to do it better. I started to research gender in education.

To ostracize

This word, such a mean word, has been in the English language since the 16th century, but it draws from an ancient Greek custom of getting rid of anyone who threatened the freedom of the people or who was simply embarrassing to the state. The word actually means a piece of pottery or bone. It was on such scraps of ceramic, shell or bone that citizens could inscribe the name of anyone they wanted to eliminate from society for ten years. The shards were anonymously dropped in a jar, counted and, provided enough people participated, the citizen with the most votes was banished with no chance of appeal. The social shunning of people who don't seem to fit, who may be 'embarrassing' to the dominant peer group, is, sadly, still a part of school and classroom communities. Not belonging, being different in some way, feeling different, or not conforming to the group's decided norms is a blueprint for being shunned, picked on, picked out, harassed and bullied. According to a 2011 National School Climate Survey in the United States, schools remain 'hostile environments for a distressing number of students' (Kosciw, Palmer and Greytak 4). It was found that 84.9% students heard the term 'gay' used in a pejorative way at school; 61.4% heard negative remarks about gender expression, including some coming from teachers and other staff at school (Wilson 84). That last comment is particularly disturbing. Another study drawn from student responses showed:

63.5% of students felt unsafe because of their sexual orientation or gender identity.
81.9% of students felt unsafe because of verbal harassment.
38% of students felt unsafe because of fear of physical harassment.
18.3% of students were physically harassed.
55.2% of students suffered cyber bullying.

60.4% of students did not report because they believed nothing would be done.
36.7% of students said nothing was done after reporting harassment.

(Ryan, Patraw and Bednar 84)

A later study in 2018 showed an increase in students suffering negative messages from peers, at school and on the Internet. Such students are twice as likely to be verbally or physically assaulted. This survey also reports that 14% of this community suffer from eating disorders, self-harm, depression and/or suicidality (Caldas 2), indicating that not much has changed in seven years. Students who feel bullied, harassed and even simply unsafe or uncomfortable are not in a place to learn and tend to avoid school altogether. 'I've been out of the closet for some time, I only go back in when the school day begins' (Hall 149). It is clear, 'teaching students to question oppressive and exclusionary systems of gender can help create environments where all children learn to understand gender in more complicated ways' (Ryan, Patraw and Bednar 85). Another engine that drove the creation of this book was the large percentage of students in this survey who stated that they did not believe adults would do anything about the harassment and, worse, a considerable percentage who said nothing was done after reporting the incident.

Something has to be done!

Drama and identity

The drama studio, with its exploration of alternative worlds, stories and people, is an ideal space where people can engage in thinking about identity – who am I? The answer to this question in a poster with a national flag, a name, a drawing of members of the family, is barely even a beginning, since identity is not something that is fixed or 'finished'; rather, it is in a constant state of 'becoming', even into adulthood and senior age. Such posters are momentary snapshots. Inevitably, a key aspect of identity will be gender identity – types of behaviour, movement, expression, clothing or appearance that may be shaped by family, society, culture, education and so on. Gender is one of the structures, or 'moulds', that shape identity, and it is a matrix of behaviours and patterns that are often forced upon us by sociocultural 'rules' or expectations. Gender identity (or gender expression) must be understood as something not necessarily linked to the assigned-at-birth sex of a person (which must also be questioned – who decides the biological sex of the new-born baby and what are the criteria?). It is also not necessarily linked to sexual preference – I express my gender as male and *therefore* I am attracted to females. The question of sexuality or sexual preference is appropriate in a drama classroom and probably belongs in health and social education.

Gender does not consist of two opposites, 'either/or' represented by two tick boxes on an application form. Instead, most gender research places gender identity on a spectrum with 'masculine' at one end and 'feminine' at the other. These represent 'traits' or behaviours, expressions and appearances traditionally associated with 'masculinity' or 'femininity' and have nothing to do with the so-called biological sex of a person. Once we have divorced these behaviours, traits, characteristics and expressions from specific body types – male and female – and as belonging to 'masculine' or 'feminine' it is possible to 'play' with all behaviours, characteristics and expressions and explore one's own personal make-up to become whole. I once removed all gender identifications from a text allocated randomly to students. A student approached me to complain that his character seemed to be motherly, caring, and he had no clue how to show this. I asked him to keep trying. After sharing classmates, he approached me again. He said, 'I've never felt that feeling before, you know, caring for someone so much you forget yourself and your own needs. Amazing'.

Identity is doing/drama is action

The existentialist Simone de Beauvoir's work, *The Second Sex* (1949), suggested one is not born a woman, but 'becomes' one, stating that being a woman is not something one 'is', but something one 'does'. De Beauvoir writes about the authority of culture that compels people to 'be a woman', for example. However, there is nothing innate in any body that 'becomes' a woman (behaves like, speaks like, appears like) that is necessarily female. De Beauvoir circumscribes the body 'as a situation', a temporary and shifting set of circumstances not related to anyone's so-called biological gender. Judith Butler expanded this idea considerably in the late 1980s and stated 'sex, gender and sexuality exist in relation to one another, so that if, for example, one is biologically female, one is expected to display "feminine" traits and . . . to desire men'; however, 'there is no necessary relationship between one's body and one's gender. In that case, it will be possible to have a designated "female" body and not to display traits generally considered feminine' (Salih 46).

In a drama context, this means that by 'doing' identities, students are engaged in the process of slowly 'becoming' themselves, on the understanding that these 'selves' are never complete works but simply ideas along the way. Judith Butler coined the term 'performativity' to encompass the sense of 'trying out' or 'trying on' gender identities in daily life. Clearly, the drama studio is not al life, but it does propose a space where 'trying out' is a central mission. Furthermore, in Judith er's term 'performativity' lies the essence of identity formation – a sense of 'doing', rather than '. One's (gender) identity is expressed in action, regardless of what one seems 'to be' (or e). 'In this sense, gender is always a doing' (Salih 50).
rocess of exploring identity in drama is echoed in Eisner:

> he arts is not only a way of creating performances and products; it is a way of
> ir lives by expanding our consciousness, shaping our dispositions, satisfying
> meaning (and) establishing contact with others. . . . Through this meaning
> understandings can emerge as it opens up the lived world of those that
> d marginalized, thus permitting new avenues and possibilities for positive
> lored. (Eisner 307)

a place of process, not product; a place of inquiry, excavation, plotting
vcle that begins the moment it ends.
Lehrstücke (Learning Plays) for young people as he believed that
evelopmental to our brains as watching one, 'the Learning Play is
o show the world as it changes (and also how it may be changed)'
cts Jesuit drama-as-education in 1700s Europe, outlined in
rmers or drama students who are engaged in the exploration
also the spectators,

he audience and performers that an audience can
igh the reflective lens of theater. A piece of theater
udience by being relevant . . . these performances
extual play within which social responsibility and

individual and communal response may be investigated, providing a momentary entrance into other worlds embodied in play and reflection. (Tomcyk 306)

About gender – Chapters 1 and 2

This is the mission of the drama teacher: to explicitly open doors and windows to allow the drama classroom to be a space where the exploration of identity is not only allowed but is something exciting and joyful. Chapter 1 offers a different kind of vocabulary for exploration, some strategies on inclusive action in the drama studio, and challenges the concept of 'safe' space. How can the drama teacher function as 'ally', as one who promotes both joy and risk of play? If you read no further than this, Chapter 1 has some general classroom management tools and tips for instant implementation of strategies to de-gender your classroom.

The children's literature offered as starting points in Chapter 2 deliberately calls for a playful, childish reading that demands curiosity, experimentation and lack of fear about what others might say. Bruno Bettelheim and Freud have analysed folk and fairy tales to unpick the workings of how identity is formed. A Freudian view of these tales shows how identity grows towards maturity, unifying the three distinct aspects of identity: the id, the ego and superego as key agents in most tales. The folk tale functions as a mirror of 'becoming'. Unsurprisingly, some of these folk tales are extremely gendered. The female princesses are passive and quiet, while male heroes are adventurous, courageous and bold. However, a simple gender switch of protagonist and/or antagonist quickly reveals much about the underlying assumptions about what 'masculine' and 'feminine' characters should or shouldn't do and thus challenges students to consider where hidden gender bias lurks. This chapter deliberately seeks to challenge the either/or binary system of gender where characters are either 'masculine' or 'feminine'. It asks who has control over the story and whose perspective drives the plot. Once the ancient epic Ramayana is turned on its head and seen from the perspective of the female protagonist, Sita, material for drama excavation is provided that addresses issues of fate, predetermination and self-realization and questions the concept of power and authority being necessarily a male domain. Folk tales and epic narratives provide a historical and oral perspective of the world in this chapter, but it also includes material for drama excavation that derives from adult fiction. Kafka's *Before the Law* looks at a more abstract view of the gendered world, by suggesting the idea of the threshold, standing at the edge of something, by an open door, unable to pass through. *Postcards from No Man's Land* pursues the idea of boundaries, hidden and real, and feelings of displacement, not belonging and feeling ostracized, while Joey, in Average Joey, uses a metaphor of wings to explore feelings of being different. Chapter 2 asks students to think about what is 'normal' and 'is it normal to not feel normal?' I also introduce some useful terms, such as the Ally, to suggest that positions of power to change minds, to have control over one's own journey towards identity, can be claimed by everyone.

Underlying the chapter is a concept contained in children's literature: this is the idea that there might be an inside world and an outside world and one's physicality may not represent the inner feelings and thoughts at all. Traditional Indian performance theory on representing emotions and presenting these with detachment to the spectator provides a useful model of how this might be achieved on the stage. The section on shapeshifters physically embodies the inner feelings onto the outer body and is an excellent metaphor to begin discussions about inner and outer perceptions of oneself. The same idea of conflict between inner and outer identity is explored through Boal's newspaper theatre which focuses on the gaps, chasms and fake information about real people and the media presentation of them. Many of the tales and stories here do not have a 'happy ending'. In fact, much of the children's literature presented in this chapter has an open end, where issues are not necessarily resolved, and this is because identity is not a closed process with a finite end. These stories, ranging in historical and geographical origin, written and told by authors old and young, are merely steppingstones or hints about how identity can be shaped. The stones may not make a path towards a specific place in the forest, but the journey is intriguing and hopefully engaging.

With gender – Chapters 4 and 5

The human body is the drama student's greatest resource. Charles Darwin was fascinated by human expression and sent out a survey of 15 questions to various missionaries across the world that contributed to his work *Expression of the Emotions in Man and Animals* in 1872. He asked questions such as

> Is astonishment expressed by the eyes and mouth being opened wide, and by the eyebrows being raised?
> When in low spirits, are the corners of the mouth depressed, and the inner corner of the eyebrows raised by that muscle which the French call the 'grief muscle'?
> When in good spirits do the eyes sparkle, with the skin a little wrinkled round and under them, and with the mouth a little drawn back at the corners? (Polhemus 77–78)

His 36 replies suggested that, indeed, these various bodily expressions of emotion were universally understood and biologically, not culturally, determined. This finding provides excellent potential for the exploration of facial expression and mask – where universally understood signs of emotion are fixed, stereotypical for all.

However, at a personal level, individuals can choose to heighten or suppress expression of gender identity. These are adjustments, shifts, nuances made by individuals to those universals of human behaviour that seem to declare the individual's personal identity, often related to masculinity and femininity, although these are almost certainly enculturated, not biological givens. In the 1970s, researchers created at least four different 'scientific' scales to measure masculine and feminine behaviour. These are the Bem Sex Role Inventory, the Personal Attributes Questionnaire, the Masculinity–Femininity Scale of the Adjective Check List and the PRF-ANDRO Scale (Mayo und Henley 97). However, the same authors found that under the age of puberty, there is little evidence to show that males and females express different kinds of nonverbal behaviour. Not a scale but a spectrum was created for gender self-assessment in 1987 (Stern, Barak and Gould), assuming there is universal understanding about what feminine and masculine behaviours look like. The authors offered a list of so-called character items linked to either femininity or masculinity. Another list of potential masculine and feminine differences looks at the way people walk and sit. For example, if the distance between the buttocks and the back of the chair is more than 10 centimetres then it is deemed 'masculine' behaviour (Burke).

A commonly cited example of stereotypical masculine and feminine behaviour is seen in the 'throwing like a girl' example. This study analysed the way males and females threw a ball and concluded that masculine and feminine gestures or actions were determined by physiological or biological differences between them. However, the reason girls did not throw as hard is that the males 'have been taught to experience space – their bodies in space – in a different way' (Noland 173). Instead of using the whole body to throw the ball as boys do, girls 'concentrate the motion in one limb, misjudge the space they can encompass, and thus fail to reach, extend, lean, stretch,

60.4% of students did not report because they believed nothing would be done.
36.7% of students said nothing was done after reporting harassment.

(Ryan, Patraw and Bednar 84)

A later study in 2018 showed an increase in students suffering negative messages from peers, at school and on the Internet. Such students are twice as likely to be verbally or physically assaulted. This survey also reports that 14% of this community suffer from eating disorders, self-harm, depression and/or suicidality (Caldas 2), indicating that not much has changed in seven years. Students who feel bullied, harassed and even simply unsafe or uncomfortable are not in a place to learn and tend to avoid school altogether. 'I've been out of the closet for some time, I only go back in when the school day begins' (Hall 149). It is clear, 'teaching students to question oppressive and exclusionary systems of gender can help create environments where all children learn to understand gender in more complicated ways' (Ryan, Patraw and Bednar 85). Another engine that drove the creation of this book was the large percentage of students in this survey who stated that they did not believe adults would do anything about the harassment and, worse, a considerable percentage who said nothing was done after reporting the incident.

Something has to be done!

Drama and identity

The drama studio, with its exploration of alternative worlds, stories and people, is an ideal space where people can engage in thinking about identity – who am I? The answer to this question in a poster with a national flag, a name, a drawing of members of the family, is barely even a beginning, since identity is not something that is fixed or 'finished'; rather, it is in a constant state of 'becoming', even into adulthood and senior age. Such posters are momentary snapshots. Inevitably, a key aspect of identity will be gender identity – types of behaviour, movement, expression, clothing or appearance that may be shaped by family, society, culture, education and so on. Gender is one of the structures, or 'moulds', that shape identity, and it is a matrix of behaviours and patterns that are often forced upon us by sociocultural 'rules' or expectations. Gender identity (or gender expression) must be understood as something not necessarily linked to the assigned-at-birth sex of a person (which must also be questioned – who decides the biological sex of the new-born baby and what are the criteria?). It is also not necessarily linked to sexual preference – I express my gender as male and *therefore* I am attracted to females. The question of sexuality or sexual preference is not appropriate in a drama classroom and probably belongs in health and social education.

Gender does not consist of two opposites, 'either/or' represented by two tick boxes on an application form. Instead, most gender research places gender identity on a spectrum, with 'masculine' at one end and 'feminine' at the other. These represent 'traits' or behaviours, expressions and appearances traditionally associated with 'masculinity' or 'femininity' and have nothing to do with the so-called biological sex of a person. Once we have divorced the idea of behaviours, traits, characteristics and expressions from specific body types – male and female – and as belonging to 'masculine' or 'feminine' it is possible to 'play' with all behaviours, traits, characteristics and expressions and explore one's own personal make-up to become 'label free'. I once removed all gender identifications from a text allocated randomly to students. A male student approached me to complain that his character seemed to be motherly, caring and kind, and he had no clue how to show this. I asked him to keep trying. After sharing the piece with classmates, he approached me again. He said, 'I've never felt that feeling before, you know, caring for someone so much you forget yourself and your own needs. Amazing'.

Identity is doing/drama is action

The existentialist Simone de Beauvoir's work, *The Second Sex* (1949), suggested one is not born a woman, but 'becomes' one, stating that being a woman is not something one 'is', but something one 'does'. De Beauvoir writes about the authority of culture that compels people to 'be a woman', for example. However, there is nothing innate in any body that 'becomes' a woman (behaves like, speaks like, appears like) that is necessarily female. De Beauvoir circumscribes the body 'as a situation', a temporary and shifting set of circumstances not related to anyone's so-called biological gender. Judith Butler expanded this idea considerably in the late 1980s and stated 'sex, gender and sexuality exist in relation to one another, so that if, for example, one is biologically female, one is expected to display "feminine" traits and . . . to desire men'; however, 'there is no necessary relationship between one's body and one's gender. In that case, it will be possible to have a designated "female" body and not to display traits generally considered feminine' (Salih 46).

In a drama context, this means that by 'doing' identities, students are engaged in the process of slowly 'becoming' themselves, on the understanding that these 'selves' are never complete works but simply ideas along the way. Judith Butler coined the term 'performativity' to encompass the sense of 'trying out' or 'trying on' gender identities in daily life. Clearly, the drama studio is not real life, but it does propose a space where 'trying out' is a central mission. Furthermore, in Judith Butler's term 'performativity' lies the essence of identity formation – a sense of 'doing', rather than 'being'. One's (gender) identity is expressed in action, regardless of what one seems 'to be' (or not to be). 'In this sense, gender is always a doing' (Salih 50).

The process of exploring identity in drama is echoed in Eisner:

> Work in the arts is not only a way of creating performances and products; it is a way of creating our lives by expanding our consciousness, shaping our dispositions, satisfying our quest for meaning (and) establishing contact with others. . . . Through this meaning making, new understandings can emerge as it opens up the lived world of those that are silenced and marginalized, thus permitting new avenues and possibilities for positive change to be explored. (Eisner 307)

The drama classroom is a place of process, not product; a place of inquiry, excavation, plotting and revision – a creative cycle that begins the moment it ends.

Brecht specifically wrote Lehrstücke (Learning Plays) for young people as he believed that performing a play can be as developmental to our brains as watching one, 'the Learning Play is essentially dynamic; its task is to show the world as it changes (and also how it may be changed)' (Willett 79). Brecht's vision reflects Jesuit drama-as-education in 1700s Europe, outlined in Chapter 4. Thus, it is not just performers or drama students who are engaged in the exploration of identity through a performance but also the spectators,

> It is within the encounter between the audience and performers that an audience can begin to see itself and the issues through the reflective lens of theater. A piece of theater can offer significant contribution to the audience by being relevant . . . these performances have the capacity to open spaces of intertextual play within which social responsibility and

and follow through in the direction of their intention' (Noland 173). Noland continues, 'As a result of years of being observed and inhibited, the female body tends to underestimate its ability to fill and traverse space' (Noland 174). Moreover, a young girl is told she must be careful 'not to get hurt, not to get dirty, not to tear her clothes, that the things she desires to do are dangerous for her. Thus, she develops a bodily timidity that increases with age' (Noland 174). Another is the example of the boardroom situation, where a female is sitting at the head of the table, in the position of power. Although she has assumed the correct proxemic position of status, she may not be in the same situation of power as a male might have been because there are other social, nonverbal cues at work (Mayo und Henley 6). In this case, spatial cues about power dominate physical cues.

Such conclusions are on the verge of becoming descriptions of masculine and feminine stereotypes. They are the external, physical cues that are accepted stereotypes of feminine and masculine behaviours even if each culture, era or individual shapes such stereotypes slightly differently. In fact, gender can be considered as a repeated stylization of the body, or a set of repeated acts. These are the cues then, the external, physical movements, gestures, ways of walking and talking that an actor may identify and explore when portraying a character of a different gender – as is the case of the male performers of female roles in Shakespeare's day in Chapter 4; in the No and Kabuki theatres of Japan and the female performers of male roles of Takarazuka in Japan and Yueju in China, outlined in Chapter 5.

Such en-gendered traits of physical movement, expression, traits, behaviour and expression can be destructive. Ray Birdwhistell explains:

> We may, however, make this generalization: in every society, before attaining membership on that society, the child must gain control of the pattern of, and be incorporated into, the communication system of the society. And, to repeat, in every society we know anything about . . . this occurs by the time the child is six years old. (Birdwhistell 7)

Furthermore,

> If his system is different from that of the group in which he grows up, he will consistently feed his parents and peers distorted information about himself and his state of mind. He will receive from the outside world information that cannot help but lead him into further distress or privacy. (Birdwhistell 16)

Thus, it is important to recognize the term *stereotyping* when looking at gender in performance. These are studied adoptions of stereotyped gesture and stance, walk and expression that an actor can 'learn' in order to represent a particular en-gendered body. Noland explains, 'it requires movement practitioners to realize to what a great extent gestures are not merely inscriptions in a metaphorical sense. Gestures literally transform the bodies that perform them' (Noland 212).

Shakespeare's motto at the Globe Theatre, 'All the world's a Playhouse', draws a neat model of theatre as a microcosm of the real world. This means that actions on stage are modelled after specific ways of moving, gesturing, behaving and speaking in the world off stage. Since actors on the public stage in Shakespeare's time were mostly male, Chapter 4 looks at ways in which the male actor portrayed feminine characteristics on stage. Specifically, English Elizabethan and Restoration acting manuals are drawn into the discussion to look at hand gestures, body stance and movement that are intended to portray specific emotions and meanings on stage. The chapter asks students to consider the stereotyping of gender in gesture, stance and behaviour and explore the power of the body to communicate on stage. Material in this chapter challenges the idea that a feminine or masculine physicality is fixed, and yet observes the conventionalization of masculine and feminine stereotypes in different periods and locations of theatre history; for example, England, Japan and China. Are concepts of 'femininity' or 'masculinity' the same over time and space? For the performer, does portraying outward signs of 'femininity' and 'masculinity' affect their inner sense of self? From questions such as these, aimed at the student as performer, the chapter also looks at the student as spectator and the question of believability. The spectator seems to know and not know that the performer is presenting a gender not their own, and this dance between knowing and not-wanting-to-know might create a sense of suspense and delight. The idea of intention is discussed in this chapter and the consequences of parody and satire through the aesthetic of camp. In this chapter, students will learn that 'camp' does not mean 'gay'; they will understand the function of stereotype and conventions in performance and observe the response and knowledge of the audience in confronting these.

Without gender – Chapters 3 and 6

On the one hand the actor is learning very specific, gendered behaviours, and, on the other hand, the actor can also be liberated from gendered behaviours entirely. The focus must then turn to physical theatre and a perception of the body that simply exists as a human species ready to express emotions, thoughts and ideas above and beyond any categorization of either masculine or feminine. This is the goal of Chapters 3 and 6. Chapter 3 on fixed mask, painted mask and half mask removes the idea of gender from facial expression entirely, corroborated by historic and contemporary research. While working with mask can remove all consideration of gender, nonetheless the rules of effective mask performance reveal an interesting and helpful concept: the role is only effective if the audience response confirms it is. This chapter contrasts stage masks and social masks and, in particular, how masks for the stage exaggerate and distort facial features to create a character. The fixed mask appears to present one emotion only, but techniques of clouding and brightening (tilting) can transform the emotion into something quite different. Students might consider their own facial expressions, the clouding or brightening of their own faces in different contexts. The mask inevitably raises questions about disguise and deception or hiding one's feelings in different contexts, like the student who is a different person at school and at home. The experience of painting the entire face as in traditional Chinese theatre is key to the concept of distortion, manipulation and 'scoring' of various biographical, emotional, characteristic traits onto a face, but does the wearing or painting of a mask over the face erase a sense of the own identity completely?

Chapter 6 focuses on physical theatre through the examples of Cunningham, Lepage and Bogart where the body is a body that has no need for any kind of gender identification. All bodies are bodies in the end, a biological species, and these theorists work with a concept of body that has no need of gender assignation. As Alan Brooks, choreographer and freelance schools dance project leader, commented, movement in life is more a question of energy:

> you notice the energy and you drop your weight, open your stride a bit differently, stoop, you make yourself a little bit bigger or smaller, you try to judge your physicality to either be . . . so threatening that you're left alone in a dangerous area or so disengaged that you are invisible. (Brooks)

Rather than gendered differences in kinds of movement, Brooks sees daily movement affected more by the context: 'There are three selves: you've got the person you've got to be at school, the person you've got to be at home and the person you've got to be on the street' (Brooks). In

Chapter 6, however, context is often removed. Students are encouraged to create a movement piece that resists not only gender but also story. The movement sequence is not a finished performance, but a snapshot of a transitory moment of shape and line shared by performer and spectator that will never be repeated. Merce Cunningham said, 'the only way to do it, is to do it', and the emphasis of this chapter is to encourage students to see that getting up and trying things out is often a more productive technique for creating a piece of work than sitting down and talking or writing about it. The chapter takes up floor patterns and topographies raised in Chapters 2 (rasa box) and 5 (the No stage) and shows how performance arts from different times and spaces can interconnect and inspire. Similarly, this chapter reflects back on the stage design of Elizabethan theatre in Chapter 4 to discuss the synthesis of all performance and production elements in creating meaning on stage. The final section of this chapter looks at traditional folk dance. Everyone in the community is invited to join in, so that the steps and moves are completely accessible to everyone. The traditional folk dance is an event that unifies and harmonizes everyone within a community for a special occasion. It has traditional male and female roles in pairs, but these can easily be transformed by the concept of Leader and Follower to become equalizing. Where the former physical movement theatres are exploratory and not formalized, the folk dance has strict rules and conventions of patterning, that can be oppositional, complementary and symmetrical. However, by the end of the dance, these rules are usually deliberately smashed as the music gets faster, dancers get dizzier and everyone collapses in a heap, laughing. The dance is inclusive; all bodies move in similar ways for similar reasons.

Do not feel obliged to read the chapters in their numerical order. Follow whatever path your compass decides, take a shortcut, backtrack, jump ahead. The ideas are suggestions, like gender itself, nonlinear. Be a magpie – take only the bits, if any, that you find sparkle.

Resources

Birdwhistell, Ray. *Kinesics and Context: Essays on Body Motion Communication*. Philadelphia: University of Pennsylvania Press, 1970.

Brooks, Alan. *Interview*. Jo Riley. February 2020.

Burke, Phyllis. *Gender Shock: Exploding the Myths of Male and Female*. New York: Anchor/Doubleday, 1996.

Caldas, Blanca. "Juxtaposing William and Graciela: Exploring Gender Nonconformity through Drama-Based Pedagogy in a Dual Language Classroom." *Composition Forum* 41. Spring 2019 (2018). https://doi.org/10.1002/tesj.420

Eisner, Elliot W. *The Arts and the Creation of the Mind*. New Haven, CT: Yale University Press, 2002.

Hall, Horace. "Teach to Reach: Addressing LGBT Youth Issues in the Classroom." *New Educator* 2 (2006): 149–157.

Johnstone, Keith. *Impro*. Methuen, 1981.

Kosciw, Joseph, Neal Palmer, and Emily Greytak. "The Effect of Negative School Climate on Academic Outcomes for LGBT Youth and the Role of In-School Supports." *Journal of School Violence* 12 (2013): 45–63.

Mayo, Clara and Nancy M. Henley. *Gender and Non-verbal Behaviour*. New York: Springer, 1981.

Noland, Carrie. *Agency and Embodiment*. Cambridge, MA: Harvard University Press, 2009.

Polhemus, Ted, ed. *The Body Reader. Social Aspects of the Human Body*. New York: Pantheon, 1978.

Ryan, Caitlin, Jasmine Patraw, and Marie Bednar. "Discussing Princess Boys and Pregnant Men, Teaching about Gender Diversity and Transgender Experiences within an Elementary School Curriculum." *LGBT Youth* 10 (2013): 83–105.

Salih, Sarah. *Routledge Critical Thinkers: Judith Butler*. London: Routledge, 2002.

Stern, Barbara B., Benny Barak, and Stephen Gould. "Sexual Identity Scale: A New Self-Assessment Measure." *Sex Roles* 17.9/10 (1987): 503–627.

Tomcyk, Patrick. "What's all the Drama? A Review of Out and Allied: An Anthology of Performance Pieces." *Journal of LGBT Youth* 13.3 (2016): 305–307.

Willett, John, ed. *Brecht on Theatre*. London: Methuen, 1987.

Wilson, Anna. "Deconstructing Homophobia through Performance: A Review of Ugly Ducklings: A National Campaign to Reduce Bullying and Harassment of Lesbian, Gay, Bisexual, Transgender and Questioning Youth." *Journal of LGBT Youth* 11 (2014): 83–89.

CHAPTER 1
Tools and equipment of discovery

As a young woman, on the verge of starting university, I found myself in Canada, in the Yukon, to be precise. Two friends and I were encouraged to hike the Chilkoot Trail from Skagway, Alaska (a little tail of Alaska on the West coast that dips into British Columbia). The trail is an ancient mountain pass created by the indigenous Tlingit people as a trade route from the coast to the interior, but the Hudson Bay Trading Company and the Klondike Goldrush dominated and controlled it from the late 1880s as a route to the Yukon gold mines. It's a five-day hike. We carried a one-man tent, two sleeping bags, some dried moose steaks, biscuits and a water bottle. It was September, so we wore jeans and t-shirts and light, canvas shoes though I later discovered that in the past, a prospector was only allowed on the trail with 1 ton of provisions to last the year. The mountain pass is stunningly beautiful. The vivid green trees; the sparkling turquoise waters; the chittering of mountain birds; the damp moss that sinks to the ankles since no one has stepped there before; the tang of wild blueberries; these sensations wrap the body in a wholesome, peaceful embrace. But the hike is also difficult, physically demanding. Echoes of the past lie at the sides of the path taken: a stove lid, an iron wheel, wires and cables, boot soles, a steam boiler, a cooking stove, parts of a piano – remnants of discarded homes that the prospectors could no longer carry forward to their tent cities and new lives. In recent years, climbers have even uncovered 50 bundles of canvas and wood 'knock down boats' 16 miles from the ocean and over 3,000 feet above sea level. We hit the snow line on the second day and were woefully underprepared, shivering, soaked and struggling to keep going in a vicious snowstorm. Canadians are rescuers, of course, so once we reached the peak between Alaska and British Columbia and stumbled into the tiny wooden hut, we were given thick slices of bread, ham and cheese, hot tea and blankets with friendly smiles. When we awoke, we were alone again, and started the trail down the other side of the mountain. We were tired, elated, deeply satisfied and relieved all at once and arrived finally back in the Yukon, at Carcross (Caribou Crossing), population 301. There was not a soul who had not heard about our journey, who could not recount how much ham and cheese we had consumed, who did not laugh at our canvas shoes and solo tent. The hike of the mad English climbers travelled ahead of us everywhere we went for many weeks. People waved at us on the streets of White Horse, calling us by name and joking about our shoes. The trail tells a story to each of those who hike it – their own, as well as the stories of all who have passed before, as

DOI: 10.4324/9781003080800-2

well as all those who will take it in future. It's not unlike a drama expedition into unknown territory. Others may have gone before, but, for us, it's new, uncharted, in our personal history. There may be some signs along the way, some artefacts, some inspirations and some struggles. But the journey is definitely worth the taking! And we will leave our mark.

Expedition preparation

Take a moment to write down the names of any explorers you can think of.

Does your list include any female explorers, such as Jeanne Boret, Ida Pfeifer or Bessie Coleman? Does your list include any explorers from outside Europe? We must arm ourselves with other, non-binary, non-Eurocentric histories. How poor in diversity is our knowledge of all those who go before us!

Luckily, we are here now together, and we shall stand in for all humanity with our own diversity. We can start the drama–gender journey with some questions, some maps, some leylines (paths between important landmarks), some cairns (stone piles that mark such sites), some tools for digging, some tools for translating and interpreting – and that bottomless rucksack of creativity that each of us carry to the drama classroom.

All drama teachers are familiar with structuring content for exploration. The most useful handbook I have found is *Structuring Drama Work* by Jonothan Neelands and Tony Goode which looks at drama conventions such as context-building action, narrative action, poetic action and reflective action. It details all the tools of devised drama, including circle of life, collective character, sound scape, hot seating, mantle of the expert, Teacher-in-Role, forum theatre, role reversal, choral work, group sculpture, space between, marking the moment, thought-tracking and many, many more. Particularly the second section, showing how to structure a starting point for learning, is very helpful. Neelands explains a process whereby identifying the content through personal and social experience moves to psychological processes where ownership of the material is established before the stage of imagining, or moving from response to action, generating meanings in a piece through atmosphere, tension, emotion and meaning (Neelands and Goode 94–104). These are all excellent techniques for 'mining' or 'excavating' material in the process of playing with identity.

A second resource that might prove useful is the glossary of terms with a range of gender vocabulary, if you are as unsure as I was about what words to use in the classroom. The glossary is compiled from several resources, but words in use are always changing and slipping over time, so I would always recommend talking to the students in your specific ensemble about 'terms of use' as you go to make sure everyone agrees on what means what. It's a joint process of discovery, and you must be prepared to throw overboard all terms that are derogatory or negative in connotation.

A third resource is the list of literature and online sites about gender in education; gender in theatre history and world theatre, mask and physical theatre included at the end of each chapter.

Basecamp - practice as learning

I am always surprised when students claim, 'I can't do that', as if acting were something that every person can do automatically, naturally without even thinking. The examples of actor training in this book, though from different historic periods and geographic locations, surely demonstrate the need for actors of all forms of theatre to practice their craft; to learn 'how to', and to keep practicing, in order that some aspects of the work finally become embedded in a body memory. In the same way that you know where to put your hand to turn on the light when entering your bedroom (you don't have to investigate first and try a variety of possibilities), this automatic response, or kinaesthetic memory, is a useful tool in the actor's armoury.

The actor's training is also cognitive – the actor is highly aware of what the body is doing and observing the doing of an action in the moment of action. All performance training requires

> a repetition of exercises over an extended amount of time and . . . neural pathways are forged with repetition, combined with attention. As we repeat an action with attention, myelin wraps around the axons of the neurons strengthening the circuit and creating the pathway for that information. Performers are trained to pay attention to their training, in detail, with consciousness; they are also trained to create, from these established pathways, different movements, actions and characters that will, in turn, re-alter neural pathways – an eternally evolving consciousness within the art form. (McCutcheon und Sellers-Young 5)

Practice and cognitive awareness or giving attention to what we are doing in the moment of doing require time and effort – it is not something that happens of itself. Thus, it must be trained.

All the theatre practices in this book require an amount of practice, if not training. This involves discipline, repetition and concentration as well as a heightened awareness of oneself. The term 'rehearsal' comes from the Old French word 'to harrow' (hercer) and describes the action of turning the earth over and over again to refine it for sowing the seed. Repetition, discipline and focus are what Bonnie Ekand describes as the embodiment of deep practice (Ekand). Deep practice requires breaking things down into smaller pieces, repeating things over and over again so that, finally, the actor can absorb it into a repertoire of automatic or memory actions. Students are often impatient, rushing to a superficial solution or movement. If the drama process is to be fulfilling, however, they should be encouraged to take time to learn and perfect their movements. It will require repetition and more repetition; as Lepage says, 'the first performance is only the first rehearsal, since the performance is never "done"'.

The ascent – a state of readiness

Just as climbers must prepare for a mountain ascent, the whole ensemble must prepare themselves for the difficult climb of making theatre together. Introduce students to the idea of a 'prepared body', one that has let go of the everyday and is in suspense, waiting, excited and focused about what is going to happen now. Eugenio Barba uses the term 'sats' to describe this kind of energy. It is an energy that is 'suspended in immobility', not like silence or stillness, although students should be silent and still. It is a stillness that contains a 'nearly ready to take action' kind of feeling. Many theatre theorists discuss this state of readiness. It is like Meyerhold's 'otkaz' or Ann Bogart's 'soft focus' – the whole body listens, is waiting, is ready to move.

Pedagogy of joy, pedagogy of risk

Besides a ready, focused approach to the drama activity, there must be a sense that everyone in the drama classroom, including the teacher, is a part of the dynamic. Bell Hooks suggests an engaged pedagogy that asks teachers to 'genuinely value everyone's presence. There must be ongoing recognition that everyone influences the classroom dynamic, that everyone contributes. These contributions are resources' (Namulundah 106). Teachers will need tact to negotiate drama tasks that deal with 'gender, failure, rupture, domestication, entrapment, sacrifice, vulnerability, and pain' (Hartley 3). The teacher is as much part of the journey as the student, and it is no surprise that Hartley links the term 'tact' with its etymological origins in 'to touch'. 'The need for trust calls for a concern for each student; it demands that the student is "seen" by the teacher and that this seeing is used to attend to their development as both a learner and a person' (Hartley 31). Hartley's book describes her teaching of trapeze skills to students at the Central School of Speech and Drama in London. Her approach is not unlike daring to take on the danger of 'gender' in the drama classroom and her observations are very useful. She says:

> It is the very character of curiosity which makes it a fundamental part of the framework I use within the classroom. I am attentive to newness, which means that I am open to receiving information on a number of levels as it comes to view. A change in breathing pattern by a student, or a memory that provokes me to offer an anecdote rather than a technical solution to the struggling student, are brought to consciousness and either attended or rejected by the teacher. These are all deviations from a set route from one place to another within my teaching, but curiosity enables me to see the individual within the frame. (Hartley 32)

Alongside tact and curiosity and attention to newness, Hartley also introduced 'consent' into her classroom practice. This ranged from a letter to parents and guardians concerning the physical risks of trapeze work to a conversation about risks with the students in person and the opportunity to ask questions, as well as a sense that at any point, the student could rescind consent. Depending on the school atmosphere it may be necessary to follow some of these formal steps. It is certainly wise to follow the general practice of making sure that students know what they are letting themselves in for with a unit in drama on gender. The students must be given some agency in their choices. The management of these choices must rest with the student. However, a unit on gender in drama should never be presented as something 'dangerous' or 'risky', implying that there are people who 'know better', or who might disapprove of or condemn such a focus. Since everyone in the space of the drama classroom at any one time is complicit in exploring gender, there is no particular goal or outcome expected from the work. The students and teachers will discover for themselves if the process has anything to offer and what it may have to offer, and this comes back to the old friend of drama teachers: trust. The teacher does not need to be a master in the skills being introduced, but the teacher does have to engage the students and fire them with curiosity. Paolo Freire argues for a pedagogy of love, yet a love that is 'armed' as if ready for battle, since it is

> driven by the feeling that it is right and dutiful to fight for the topic, to denounce and announce aspects and discoveries encountered and to continue provoking and challenging students to keep going even when the topic feels weird, odd, difficult or embarrassing. (Hartley 121)

This feels quite like the 'sats' energy of anticipation mentioned above.

Finally, and as always in a drama class, in contradiction to all the above, the teacher must sense when it is time to 'walk away'. Keeping distance from the student work and allowing it to develop in its own way, knowing that even if the formal drama assessment work may not reach a specifically predefined criterion, it is more than possible that the student is learning important things in discussions with friends and family outside the classroom, and that may be just as important as what's happening under the teacher's guidance.

Water rest - the safe space

Borrowing from Jonothan Neelands' four key conditions of making theatre (Neelands, Beginning Drama 11–14), I wonder if I can adapt the list of priorities in drama teaching so that the challenging creative environment, the space, comes first. All the world may very well be represented on the microcosm of the theatre stage, but every drama classroom is also microcosm of the world as well. The participants in the classroom come from different places both literally and psychologically and must learn to get along with each other in collaborative effort if there is to be a creative outcome. Everyone teaching drama talks about the studio as a 'safe space' that respects and tolerates difference. Whether the space is a classroom with tables pushed back or a darkened fit-for-purpose theatre studio, the term 'safe space' implies more than a physically safe environment.

Safety is one of the base foundations of Maslow's Hierarchy of Needs that leads to self-fulfilment, which, in this case, I will assume to be the precondition of being able *to dare to create*. Thus, self-fulfilment, achieving one's full potential and creativity, is predicated on physical and mental safety, when bodily needs (food, water,) and psychological needs (care, rest) are met. Clearly, physical safety in a drama classroom is important. Hunter suggests four areas of safety. The first is physical – the environment (lighting, heating); the second is social safety (what happens in Vegas stays in Vegas); the third is familiarity and comfort within the group of participants; and the fourth is the extent to which the space facilitates the creativity of all participants (Barrett). A 'safe space' in the drama classroom might also mean a place where offensive language, and behaviour is explicitly controlled with a sign outside the door that says, 'In this room we will not tolerate the use of any words or actions that put people down because of race, religion, gender, sexual orientation, or disability'. It might be a coded sign system of rainbow stickers, indicating that this classroom is a safe space supportive of all students like the materials offered by the GLSEN safe space kit and other support organizations. Or does it lie with classroom management, teacher response and action when language and behaviour in the classroom is offensive? Or, is the teacher equally bound up in their own privileges of colour, status, gender, nationality, ethnicity and so on? Behaviours that interfere with learning such as name-calling, tone of voice, sarcasm, interrupting and aggressive body language are things that do not belong in a classroom. This might suggest that a 'safe space' is actually the lack of something negative rather than a presence of something positive (Barrett 12). In this sense, a safe space can actually reinforce the current power structures between participants so that, to succeed, the teacher must account for context and time, place and manner of infringement before deciding whether to act punitively or not. There is a danger that the term 'safe space' can sound like a 'security blanket' to cover important and challenging issues in life. Furthermore, it is important to ask the question 'for whom is it safe?' Students and teachers arrive in the drama classroom with a wide range of beliefs, languages and cultures 'acting like nation-states in which they're consciously and fully immersed, whether or not they explicitly inform us of that' (Caldas 4). Students and teachers may already have raised their castle walls against attack!

In a study conducted by Holley and Steiner regarding characteristics that students felt contributed to a safe learning environment, the majority of students declared it was the responsibility of the instructor to ensure participant safety (Holley and Steiner). The instructor should be seen to be non-judgemental or unbiased (Barrett 6). The concept of 'safe space' suggests that dangerous, provocative, challenging ideas and thoughts will not be let loose here. Instead, the teacher might issue a 'trigger warning' before beginning a particular topic. However, as early as 1998, Robert Boostrom suggested that education should be neither safe nor comfortable. Instead, he felt that students should be criticized and challenged (Boostrom). In the context of gender studies, 'safe space' has come to mean an environment with clear boundaries, such as counsellor offices, community centres and other meeting places, where everyone can feel safe from physical and emotional harm and can gain a sense of comfort and belonging and the freedom to express themselves (Ziv). The dilemma here is that a space that allows people to behave and speak as they wish must also permit access to new ideas and practices, to make mistakes and ask questions, which seems mutually exclusive.

In the drama context, a safe space is more than this. According to Hunter, 'safe space' must include the creative potential for tension and risk. Therefore, a safe space for drama teachers is more than just a preparation to perform – it is 'a space of messy negotiations that allow individual and group actions of representation to occur' (Lambert 22). The safe space of the drama classroom is an 'open space' (Gallagher) which allows relationships and interactions to flourish. We might not be able to list or map what 'goes into' making a safe space in the drama classroom, but we all seem to recognize it when we see it. A so-called safe space might be safe for some and not for others, depending on the social-cultural-gender-racial-ethnic mix of the group concerned. A space that guarantees dignity of those within it might protect intellectual safety, quashing the impulse to speak up, deny, negate or challenge. A safe space might be a space where difficult, challenging or thought-provoking challenges are never raised, for fear of offending, or upsetting someone, as if the class was composed of 'snowflakes'. So, are there other models of space that might be useful for our drama–gender expedition?

Nomad space and sedentary space

In investigating the sense of 'becoming' in terms of identity, Deleuze and Guattari devised a metaphor of territory: staying within one's familiar territory; moving out of one's territory (de-territorialization); and incorporating the new aspects of the new territory into the stable identity (re-territorialization). Different kinds of space allow for these processes. Smooth space, or nomad space, allows for fluid, unfixed and exploratory action and reflects the process of de-territorialization where everyone is different and curious about what's out there (cited in Lambert 117). It has a flowing energy unhindered by obstacles. The opposite is striated (striped, streaked) or sedentary space which is represented by rules and regulations that constrict movement, where everyone is the same or uniform. Striated space would include rules of gender that should be strictly observed. Smooth or nomad space does not necessarily mean a space with no physical obstacles just as striated or sedentary space does not mean a classroom with desks and chairs. Smooth or nomad space allows psychological movement, or flow, where there is a freedom of intellectual curiosity with no boundaries or rules. Smooth space would allow for exploration of identities without needing to be confined to gender boundaries set by social or peer norms, for example. Continuing this thinking, Tim Ingold writes that 'lives are led not inside places but through, around, to and from them, from and to places elsewhere' (Caldas).

A space of flow

Mihaly Csikszentmihalyi, American psychologist, also wrote about the sense of 'flow' being crucial to creativity (Csikszentmihalyi), not unlike Deleuze and Guattari's idea of 'nomad space'.

Csikszentmihalyi noticed that people engaged in challenging activities experience a sense of deep and effortless concentration that he calls 'flow' experiences – key to understanding this concept is the idea of 'doing' of being an active part in the creative process. This brings the passive 'safe space', the 'negative space' of something missing closer to an active safe space where 'doing' or 'being' is the key.

Civil space

This idea was sparked by Robert Boostrom who argued strongly that students needed to be exposed to different viewpoints, perspectives and beliefs and learn to manage conflict and criticism. He proposed a 'classroom agora' or 'classroom as congress'. This idea was further elaborated by other scholars (Flensner and Von der Lippe) to include a sense of civility, since freedom of speech is a fundamental human right and students and teachers should be able to express their views and respect the dignity of everyone else's views as well. It sounds a little too political for the drama classroom, but the concept holds.

Brave or unsafe space

Robert Boostrom moved even further and proposed the concept of 'brave space', suggesting that bravery was needed to relinquish old habits and perspectives and be open to the world and oneself in new ways – which is the mission of drama in the curriculum. Arao and Clemens argue that 'authentic learning about diversity and social justice requires that the students and the teachers are willing to put themselves at risk' (Arao and Clemens). The term 'brave' encourages an active and positive sense of courage – something you can do something about – rather than a somewhat passive illusion of 'being safe'. Adhering to this idea, James Arnt Aune claimed, 'classrooms should be unsafe spaces' (Stob). Boostrom firmly states that criticism is key to growth,

> When everyone's voice is accepted and no one's voice can be criticized, then no one can grow … that we need to hear other voices to grow is certainly true, but we also need to be able to respond to those voices, to criticize them, to challenge them, to sharpen our own perspectives through the friction of dialogue. (cited in Barrett 8)

Contact zone, neutral space or communities of disagreement

In teaching queer studies at Oberlin College, Jan Cooper came across another metaphor for the space of exploration – the 'Contact zone'. This should describe a space (not literal) where all participants can come into contact with all kinds of possibilities. The zone was like Switzerland – it was to be a neutral space where 'classes, discussions, and student encounters with texts occur'. It was intended as a 'zone of coalitioning ideas' (Cooper). However, this term feels too military, or at least too political for the drama classroom. Building on it is a term developed by Iverson in 2018 – 'communities of disagreement', which is defined as 'a group with identity claims, consisting of people with different opinions, who find themselves engaged in a common process, in order to solve shared problems or challenges' (Flensner and Von der Lippe).

Before the drama can start, both teachers and students clearly need to define their terms of engagement. What kind of space shall this exploration take place in? I would strongly recommend discussing some of these terms with the students – we're all in this together!

The cliffhanger – a supportive community

The same research that uncovered severe gender harassment and bullying in schools also found that schools that offered Gay Straight Alliances, or allowed students to run such groups, promoting a safer climate, generally had more success in combating prejudice. Safe zones, clubs and LGBTQ+ education in health and social classes were instrumental in effecting positive change in the dominant school climate (Pynter and Tubbs). However, the presence of such alliances in schools, while it decreased the incidents of gender harassment and bullying, did not improve student self-esteem or educational outcomes of students who felt bullied or harassed. Remaining silent was found to be extremely distressing to the whole student community. The key factor in changing how students felt about themselves at school was, of course, the way adults in their lives responded to their issues. 'The strongest positive influence . . . was having supportive adults at school' (Kosciw, Palmer and Greytak 58). These adults must be askable and approachable. Alongside school-based alliances for students, there are also several organizations such as PFLAG that support parents and friends who will extend the atmosphere in school to the home and world outside the school gates. Such alliances can be very helpful when the home environment is less accepting than in school (Keck und Perry) and are vital in recruiting allies.

Teacher as ally

An ally is deemed 'a person who is a member of the dominant or majority group who works to end oppression in his or her personal and professional life through the support of and as an advocate with, and for the oppressed population', and this person can be 'instrumental in effecting positive change in the dominant culture' (Kosciw, Palmer and Greytak 122). Action is the key responsibility of an ally – by raising their voice against gender issues. In the classroom, a teacher as ally can change the dynamics of the ensemble by being educated themselves on matters concerning gender; by being seen to help to educate others on gender issues, by getting involved in activities and creating an environment in class where students learn to understand gender in more complicated ways. A teacher as ally is a teacher who listens and cares about where the answer might be coming from in a specifically caring pedagogy,

> where what the student says matters, right or wrong and . . . where the teacher pushes gently for clarification and interpretation. The teacher is not seeking the answer but the involvement of the student. . . . The student is infinitely more important than the subject matter. (Noddings 176)

It also means being aware of practices that might be embedded or institutionalized over time that need urgent review. For example, using material in the classroom that stereotypes male and female behaviours, appearance and expression without drawing attention to the stereotyping. Or, being closed to mixed sports teams if desired by the students; dismissing students to watch male athletics matches but not female ones; punishing male students by having them join the female students; calling out 'boys and girls' or having them line up in their assigned gender roles; making single-gendered groups of boys or girls compete against each other in any discipline – in fact, to raise gender in any activity students are engaged in where gender is actually irrelevant. A further action that can be undertaken by teacher as ally is to check the school handbook. Clear policies must be in place that lay out what happens when gender harassment or gender bullying has taken place. Finally, the teacher as ally may also have the responsibility of educating colleagues and administration personnel in the school.

The panorama – some easy ways to be inclusive today

If you read no further in this book, here are some quick ideas to include everyone in the ensemble.

Replace gender pronouns such as 'she', 'he', 'her', 'his' with 'the', 'they', 'their' or a student name in everything you say: 'Looks like someone left their jacket on the chair'; 'I asked the costume designer and they told me . . .'; 'let's see how Terry reacts to the conflict'.

Include everyone by making sure to speak to every single person in the room by using a pot of sticks with names on to call on students, or an online randomizing name generator. This ensures unbiased grouping and questioning without subconscious prejudice. Start a practice of entrance/exit questions. As each student leaves/enters the classroom they must answer an open question you set about learning today; about someone who impressed them or about themselves. It must be a goal that every student has spoken to the teacher at least once every class.

When speaking to the ensemble as a whole, avoid gendered group terms such as 'guys', 'boys', 'girls' instead favouring 'friends', 'everyone', 'wildcats' (or school mascot), 'students'. Encourage the ensemble to use these terms when speaking to each other in collaborative work.

When choosing stimuli for devised work, or teacher in role units, choose character names that are gender-neutral such as, Alex, Chris, Jo, Cameron, Charlie, AJ, Terry, Riley, Taylor . . . alternatively, work with A, B, C and so on.

When generating devised work adapt Brecht's model of Verfremdung by avoiding the individualization of characters. Brecht's characters are largely defined by their roles, jobs or actions: Teacher, Worker, Guardian, Child, Student, Parent, Victim, Oppressor, Rebel, the Lonely One, the Fearful One, the Shy One and so on.

When distributing published texts for exploration, include postmodern play texts with no designations of character. Works by Martin Crimp, Caryl Churchill, Roland Schimmelpfennig, Patrick Marber, Marius von Mayenburg and Mark Ravenhill frequently do not designate character speech and instead use a hyphen when the speaker changes. This allows for an open gender interpretation of character.

In distributing text extracts for dialogue or pairs work, replace character names with A or B and remove any other gender markers in the text such as 'mother', father, 'she' or 'he', observing the pronoun rules above. Explain to the students that you have done this, and why you have done this. A text that explores the relationship between a mother and daughter can be interpreted by any person of any gender or generation.

In choosing plays for performance or curriculum study include some famous queer theatre artists and explicitly state their alliances. For example, Tennessee Williams, Oscar Wilde, Edward Albee, Tony Kushner, Howard Brenton, Robert Wilson, Noel Coward, Joe Orton, Aphra Behn, Harvey Fierstein, Federico Garcia Lorca, Jean Genet, Nikolai Gogol, Bernard-Marie Koltès, Robert LePage, Alan Bennett, among so many others. Look to the chapters in this book to include some non-Western models.

The descent – words can never hurt me

On this journey to discover gender perspectives in drama, if you are like me, you were very much about the topic before you start. And that's hopefully why you picked up

But you don't need to know anything before you start – it's quite all right to make the journey alongside your students, as I did, learning together and making mistakes together. My first approach was to collate all the different terms and words I would need to deliver a gender drama unit. I quickly realized that language, being a live form, shifts and changes; it also changes between English speakers according to their age, location, culture and learning and if you are in an international environment then it is even more important to find terms from other languages too. Still, a vocabulary list is not a bad place to start, and that's why there are some suggestions in the glossary. But it doesn't need to be dutifully learnt before the action begins. Instead, these are tools for conversations in the classroom with the students. The students will have their own words and terms for the subject, and it is important to let everyone have their say even if there is no definitive agreement. If students raise negative and offensive terms, the teacher as ally will be able to explain calmly that there is no place for these.

Archaeology and cartography

Each of the chapters in this book offers some background information, theory or explanation of a theatre form – children's stories, mask, Elizabethan and Restoration drama, Japanese No theatre, Kabuki and Takarazuka, Chinese Yueju and Physical theatre. There is no imperative to read or follow the chapters in any order whatsoever. Moreover, there is no attempt to offer curriculum or assessment objectives, since you are most familiar with how these work at your school and you are the expert. Change the material to fit your needs. I also urge you to use your favourite warm-ps and exercises to keep activity, focus and trust-work flowing alongside the gender excavations. You know the theatre forms suggested in this book very well already, so the introductions I am /iding here are very superficial and I am expecting that you will easily be able to source more 'ed and thorough information in print and online to support the work as needed. I have tried the key aspect of each theatre form to a series of lesson ideas which I call 'excavations' ense of an archaeological dig. The archaeologist locates clues as to the possible area igation by a kind of aerial reconnaissance, a distant overview. Then, the archaeologist some preliminary marking of the territory and very slowly starts to uncover the layers of ase the secret treasure inside. The excavation is sometimes painstaking, sometimes it it does require more than one visit to the site. The archaeologist must uncover e process of sifting, shovelling and cleaning through the layers, and it is a time- ess before the various artefacts can be recorded, reassembled and associated provide meaning. It is dirty work, physical work, sometimes repetitive; sometimes ried there, and the archaeologist has to move to another location and try again. n' seemed to encompass the drama work of exploration much better than exploration'.

ve of gender in the drama classroom also offered me a different view of an de la Cosa was a Spanish mapmaker, who was the navigation master s' voyage to the Americas in 1492. He charted a first map after the next a second map in 1498 and a third, in 1499, when he made the voyage lis final map of 1500 is known as the Map of the World, yet it certainly admire the tenacity and courage of this man who travelled several times ought back charts that became increasingly accurate yet never quite that his approach is an apt metaphor for mapping, what is for me, a ma. It is important to change the classroom vocabulary and find new are attempting. I have used the phrases Survey the terrain, Set the compass, Reset the compass for moments where students might, in pairs or groups or whole class, stop and consider where they are now and where to go next. The hated word 'reflection' must be eradicated from drama classrooms, since students associate this word with parrot-like responses about 'things I have learned' and 'things I can do better' that they believe the teacher wants to hear. 'Reflection' seems to imply there is a 'right' answer and the aim of the writing is to show whether or not you reached it. Thus, I have replaced this term with the cartographer's term, 'reckoning', which is the ability to estimate roughly where you are at any one moment in time. It's like an educated guess, bearing in mind certain fixed points or known locations. It allows for adjustment to continue beyond the moment of thinking about things, since the journey is not ending here. A performance is not the end of a process in drama. A reckoning allows me to say, 'this is where I think I am at the moment', and it allows me to posit 'I wonder how things will look different tomorrow'. A reckoning is also an oral act to be shared with others who may be on the same ship or other seas entirely. In speaking it, I am also erasing it, because the moment of verbalization is also the moment everything shifts again and that's fine, because a reckoning looks forward to what might possibly come next and how it might draw from where it is now, whereas a reflection stops the process, and merely looks back to what has been.

I hope that teachers and students who come after me will continue to improve and change the vocabulary, keep digging and discovering. Because from where I stand . . . this is how I see it, for now.

Resources

Arao, B. and K. Clemens. "From Safe Spaces to Brave Spaces: A New Way to Frame Dialogue around Diversity." *The Art of Effective Facilitation: Reflections from Social Justice Educators*. Ed. L.M. Landreman. Sterling: Stylus, 2013. 135–150.

Barrett, Betty. "Is 'Safety' Dangerous? A Critical Examination of the Classroom as Safe Space." *The Canadian Journal for the Scholarship of Teaching and Learning* 1.1 (2010). http://dx.doi.org/10.5206/-cjsotl-rcacea.2010.1.9

Boostrom, Robert. "'Safe Spaces': Reflections on an educational Metaphor." *Journal of Curriculum Studies* 30.4 (1998): 397–408.

Caldas, Blanca. "Juxtaposing William and Graciela: Exploring Gender Nonconformity through Drama-Based Pedagogy in a Dual Language Classroom." *Composition Forum* 41.Spring 2019 (2018): 1–13

Cooper, Jan. "Queering the Contact Zone." *JAC* 24.1 (2004): 23–45.

Csikszentmihaly, Mihaly. *Flow: The Psychology of Optimal Experience*. New York: Harper Collins, 2009.

Ekand, Bonnie. "Embodying Deep Practice: A Pedagogical Approach to Actor Training." *Embodied Consciousness and Performance Technologies*. Eds. J.R. McCutcheon and B. Sellers-Young. London: Palgrave Macmillan, 2013: 46–56

Flensner, Karin and Marie Von der Lippe. "Being Safe from What and Safe for Whom? A Critical Discussion of the Conceptual Metaphor of 'Safe Space'." *Intercultural Education* 30 (2019): 275–288.

Gallagher, K. "Contesting Space and Power through Digital Drama Research: Colonial Histories, Postcolonial Interrogations." *Caribbean Quarterly* 53.1–2 (2007): 115–126.

GLSEN. *The Safe Space Kit*. New York, NY: GLSEN, 2016.

Hartley, Jessica Ruth. *Guided Practices in Facing Danger*. London: Central School of Speech and Drama PhD thesis, 2013.

Holley, Lynn and Sue Steiner. "Safe Space: Student Perspectives on Classroom Environment." *Journal of Social Work and Education* 41 (2005): 49–64.

Keck, Andy and David Perry. "Challenging Heteronormativity: Creating a Safe and Inclusive Environment for LGBTQ Students." *Journal of School Violence* 17 (2018): 227–243.

Kosciw, Joseph, Neal Palmer, and Emily Greytak. "The Effect of Negative School Climate on Academic Outcomes for LGBT Youth and the Role of in School Supports." *Journal of School Violence* 12 (2013): 45–63.

Lambert, Kirsten. *More than Princess Girls and 'Grrr' Heterosexual Dudes: An Exploration of Space, Text, Performativity, Gender and Becoming in Senior Secondary Drama Classrooms.* Murdoch University PhD thesis, 2017.

McCutcheon, Jade Rosina and Barbara Sellers-Young, *Embodied Consciousness Performance Technologies.* London: Palgrave Macmillan, 2013.

Namulundah, Florence. *Bell Hooks' Engaged Pedagogy. A Transgressive Education for Critical Consciousness.* Westport, CT: Bergin and Garvey, 1998.

Neelands, Jonothan. *Beginning Drama 11–14.* London: Routledge, 2013.

Neelands, Jonothan and Tony Goode. *Structuring Drama Work: A Handbook of Available Forms in Theatre and Drama.* Cambridge: Cambridge University Press, 1990.

Noddings, Nel. *Caring. A Feminine Approach to Ethics and Moral Education.* Berkeley: University of California Press, 1984.

Pynter, Kerry and Nancy Tubbs. "Safe Zones: Creating LGBT Safe Space Ally Programs." *Journal of LGBT Youth* 5.1 (2007): 121–132.

Stob, Paul. "No Safe Space: James Arnt Aune and the Controversial Classroom." *Rhetoric and Public Affairs* 16.3 (2013): 555–566.

Ziv, Amalia. "Questioning Safe Space in the Classroom: Reflections on Pedagogy, Vulnerability and Sexual Explicitness." *Borderlands e journal* 17.1 (2018): 1–16 taken place. Finally, the teacher as ally may also have the responsibility of educating colleagues and administration personnel in the school.

The panorama – some easy ways to be inclusive today

If you read no further in this book, here are some quick ideas to include everyone in the ensemble.

Replace gender pronouns such as 'she', 'he', 'her', 'his' with 'the', 'they', 'their' or a student name in everything you say: 'Looks like someone left their jacket on the chair'; 'I asked the costume designer and they told me . . .'; 'let's see how Terry reacts to the conflict'.

Include everyone by making sure to speak to every single person in the room by using a pot of sticks with names on to call on students, or an online randomizing name generator. This ensures unbiased grouping and questioning without subconscious prejudice. Start a practice of entrance/ exit questions. As each student leaves/enters the classroom they must answer an open question you set about learning today; about someone who impressed them or about themselves. It must be a goal that every student has spoken to the teacher at least once every class.

When speaking to the ensemble as a whole, avoid gendered group terms such as 'guys', 'boys', 'girls' instead favouring 'friends', 'everyone', 'wildcats' (or school mascot), 'students'. Encourage the ensemble to use these terms when speaking to each other in collaborative work.

When choosing stimuli for devised work, or teacher in role units, choose character names that are gender-neutral such as, Alex, Chris, Jo, Cameron, Charlie, AJ, Terry, Riley, Taylor . . . alternatively, work with A, B, C and so on.

When generating devised work adapt Brecht's model of Verfremdung by avoiding the individualization of characters. Brecht's characters are largely defined by their roles, jobs or actions: Teacher, Worker, Guardian, Child, Student, Parent, Victim, Oppressor, Rebel, the Lonely One, the Fearful One, the Shy One and so on.

When distributing published texts for exploration, include postmodern play texts with no designations of character. Works by Martin Crimp, Caryl Churchill, Roland Schimmelpfennig, Patrick Marber, Marius von Mayenburg and Mark Ravenhill frequently do not designate character speech and instead use a hyphen when the speaker changes. This allows for an open gender interpretation of character.

In distributing text extracts for dialogue or pairs work, replace character names with A or B and remove any other gender markers in the text such as 'mother', father, 'she' or 'he', observing the pronoun rules above. Explain to the students that you have done this, and why you have done this. A text that explores the relationship between a mother and daughter can be interpreted by any person of any gender or generation.

In choosing plays for performance or curriculum study include some famous queer theatre artists and explicitly state their alliances. For example, Tennessee Williams, Oscar Wilde, Edward Albee, Tony Kushner, Howard Brenton, Robert Wilson, Noel Coward, Joe Orton, Aphra Behn, Harvey Fierstein, Federico Garcia Lorca, Jean Genet, Nikolai Gogol, Bernard-Marie Koltes, Robert LePage, Alan Bennett, among so many others. Look to the chapters in this book to include some non-Western models.

The descent – words can never hurt me

On this journey to discover gender perspectives in drama, if you are like me, you won't know very much about the topic before you start. And that's hopefully why you picked up this book!

But you don't need to know anything before you start – it's quite all right to make the journey alongside your students, as I did, learning together and making mistakes together. My first approach was to collate all the different terms and words I would need to deliver a gender drama unit. I quickly realized that language, being a live form, shifts and changes; it also changes between English speakers according to their age, location, culture and learning and if you are in an international environment then it is even more important to find terms from other languages too. Still, a vocabulary list is not a bad place to start, and that's why there are some suggestions in the glossary. But it doesn't need to be dutifully learnt before the action begins. Instead, these are tools for conversations in the classroom with the students. The students will have their own words and terms for the subject, and it is important to let everyone have their say even if there is no definitive agreement. If students raise negative and offensive terms, the teacher as ally will be able to explain calmly that there is no place for these.

Archaeology and cartography

Each of the chapters in this book offers some background information, theory or explanation of a theatre form – children's stories, mask, Elizabethan and Restoration drama, Japanese No theatre, Kabuki and Takarazuka, Chinese Yueju and Physical theatre. There is no imperative to read or follow the chapters in any order whatsoever. Moreover, there is no attempt to offer curriculum or assessment objectives, since you are most familiar with how these work at your school and you are the expert. Change the material to fit your needs. I also urge you to use your favourite warm-ups and exercises to keep activity, focus and trust-work flowing alongside the gender excavations.

You know the theatre forms suggested in this book very well already, so the introductions I am providing here are very superficial and I am expecting that you will easily be able to source more detailed and thorough information in print and online to support the work as needed. I have tried to link the key aspect of each theatre form to a series of lesson ideas which I call 'excavations' in the sense of an archaeological dig. The archaeologist locates clues as to the possible area for investigation by a kind of aerial reconnaissance, a distant overview. Then, the archaeologist engages in some preliminary marking of the territory and very slowly starts to uncover the layers of soil that encase the secret treasure inside. The excavation is sometimes painstaking, sometimes bulldozing, but it does require more than one visit to the site. The archaeologist must uncover meaning in the process of sifting, shovelling and cleaning through the layers, and it is a time-consuming process before the various artefacts can be recorded, reassembled and associated with each other to provide meaning. It is dirty work, physical work, sometimes repetitive; sometimes there is nothing buried there, and the archaeologist has to move to another location and try again. The term 'excavation' seemed to encompass the drama work of exploration much better than 'exercise', or indeed 'exploration'.

The new perspective of gender in the drama classroom also offered me a different view of the world in general. Juan de la Cosa was a Spanish mapmaker, who was the navigation master on Christopher Columbus' voyage to the Americas in 1492. He charted a first map after the next voyage in 1493. He drew a second map in 1498 and a third, in 1499, when he made the voyage with Amerigo Vespucci. His final map of 1500 is known as the Map of the World, yet it certainly was not very complete. I admire the tenacity and courage of this man who travelled several times to the New World and brought back charts that became increasingly accurate yet never quite complete or finished. I find that his approach is an apt metaphor for mapping, what is for me, a New World of gender in drama. It is important to change the classroom vocabulary and find new words to describe what we are attempting. I have used the phrases Survey the terrain, Set the

CHAPTER 2

About gender - seeking identity

Being curious about yourself and your place in the world is a great place to start a drama.

My family loved books. I was not a strong reader, but luckily for me, my mother admired illustration and so there were editions of *Alice in Wonderland*, and the dark stories of the *Brothers Grimm* illustrated by Arthur Rackham on the shelves and, something that caught my eye more than even this: *The Arabian Nights*, illustrated by Edmund Dulac (childish excitement: he must be French!). Later, my mother took me along to a deserted old house to retrieve the personal belongings of a great aunt who had recently died. She was the daughter of the owner of an engineering firm in Singapore and had lived in Asia most of her life. Among rusty pill boxes in a corner cupboard, I found a little wooden model of two Chinese men sawing at a log that moved if you jiggled it about. The books *Little Plum* by Rumer Godden; *Tikki Tikki Tembo* by Arlene Mosel; an embroidered kimono in the dressing-up box – looking back on my childhood, I think there were many signs that led me to China, and they had been there all along, only I didn't know it till I looked back.

In my childhood home, we had visitors and exchange students from all over Europe, America and Australia, even Japan. I grew up struggling to speak French and German with several of them and loved watching their hands as the pen covered the page with black squiggles and signs of mystery whose meaning I couldn't guess. I thought my childhood was a kaleidoscope infused with people and things that were different from me. It pushed me to seek difference, to try out different things, to 'be' different people and speak different languages. To ask, 'why is that different' and 'how does it feel'?

These are the questions that exist in the drama classroom; it's a place where childhood curiosity for the world around us and within us can be let free. Who am I and how does it feel? Who could I be next and how would that feel? Keith Johnstone, in his book on improvisation, says that he lost his sense of curiosity and play as he grew older, 'everything started getting grey and dull'; he said that education could be a 'destructive process' only driving young people to 'get it right' (K. Johnstone 18). So, he set about to find the colours of childhood again and rediscovered the power of play, the joy of letting go, trying out and trying on.

This chapter will look at children's literature – stories of people and things far removed from us as a way of looking inside ourselves. They are stories of humankind, tales of people and events we cannot know ourselves but yet contain human truths and models for us to learn about the possible ways of the world and our places within it. Some of the stories have been around

DOI: 10.4324/9781003080800-3

for centuries; some are newer, but things that are strange to us in time or place can spark new thoughts, new languages (mental and physical) and new ways of being.

Stories and identity

Freudian psychologist Bruno Bettelheim (1903–1990) proposed the importance of Fairy Tales to every person's development and understanding of identity (Bettelheim). He suggested that stories 'have great psychological meaning for children of all ages, both girls and boys, irrespective of the age and sex of the story's hero . . . they facilitate changes in identification as the child deals with different problems' (Bettelheim 17). Bettelheim felt that by sharing stories with children, the adult was giving a vital demonstration that the child's inner experiences were worthwhile and legitimate, perhaps even 'real' and that therefore the child was equally 'real and important' to the surrounding family and world (Bettelheim 62). The drama teacher is in a prime position to keep offering stories to the ensemble. One cannot know which particular story will appeal to which child, at which stage in their development, or thought, so it is important to keep sharing, keep offering multiple story types in the drama classroom. Moreover, the process of curriculum drama demands response, action, reflection, further action; it insists that internal processes of the story are externalized into action; it allows the players to linger over a story and to dive deeply into the story's offerings in terms of how they feel about themselves and their experience of the world.

> In order to master the psychological problems of growing up – overcoming narcissistic disappointments, oedipal dilemmas, sibling rivalries; becoming able to relinquish childhood dependencies; gaining a feeling of selfhood and of self-worth, and a sense of moral obligation – a child needs to understand what is going on within the conscious self so that they can also cope with that which goes on in the unconscious. (Bettelheim 6–7)

In this chapter, I will look stories from Grimm's folk tales, Greek myths, children's literature from the UK and India, as well as contemporary children's books dealing with gender explicitly. The non-realistic nature of these stories 'is an important device, because it makes obvious that the fairy tales' concern is not useful information about the external world, but inner processes taking place in an individual' (Bettelheim 25). The stories around us and from around the world help us explore identity.

A story can be excavated on different levels:

1. A simple **metaphorical interpretation** of a well-known story might be that when Little Red Riding Hood is swallowed by the wolf, it mirrors the fear of night/darkness forever devouring the day/light; winter replacing summer, a god swallowing a sacrificial victim.
2. It may suggest a **developmental model**. Hans drops breadcrumbs and succumbs to greed in the witch's house, while the girl, Gretel, saves them, promoting a feminine trait of 'care' in young adolescence (Zipes). The tale suggests their desire to remain children, to be looked after by their parents, even though it's time for them to discover the world outside. The story is a metaphor for the next phase of life.
3. A story may be an **enactment of a fantasy world**. Children do not see objects as different from living things, so it is not unexpected that inanimate objects or animals speak, nor is it surprising that they speak back to the child about their inner fears and desires, just as the child 'talks for' the favourite cuddle toy – such dialogue is the fundamental premise of drama.
4. It may suggest the **possibility of perpetual transformation** and change, unlike super-hero stories where the superpowers are put aside at the end of the story and the hero returns to a 'normal' existence and the experience is 'put away'.

In all cases, stories contribute to different ways of exploring emerging identities. In this chapter, I have selected stories for the drama classroom that promote:

1. **Perspective shift** – by changing the gender of a key role in the story
2. **Shapeshifters** – changing the physical shape of being to explore identity
3. **Being invisible** – the feeling of being no one, an isolated individual that doesn't fit
4. **Breaking out** – mirrors/windows/doors as opportunities for self-discovery
5. **Integration of an identity** (for now) – acceptance and tolerance of oneself
6. **Recognition of 'other'** – real-life examples of people and situations

Resources

Bettelheim, Bruno. *The Uses of Enchantment. The Meaning and Importance of Fairy Tales.* London: Thames and Hudson, 1976.

Johnstone, Keith. *Impro.* London: Methuen, 1981. 18.

Zipes, Jack. *Don't Bet on the Prince. Contemporary Feminist Fairy Tales in North America and England.* New York: Routledge, 2012.

Shifting the perspective – part 1

PETER RABBIT

The Tale of Peter Rabbit (Potter) is about being greedy, selfish and taking risks. It's about realizing the consequences of actions – you reap what you sow. It is also about civilization and learning. By insisting that Peter wear a jacket and shoes (become socialized), Mrs Rabbit restricts his actions and nearly gets him killed (Nodelman). Indeed, the tale is also about rejecting maternal authority and trying to find one's own way in the world outside the family home. It's also about loss – lost shoes, lost fathers and husbands and lost rabbit pie. And finally, it's a tale about finding a tail – a young male finding his identity as an adult male.

Synopsis

Peter Rabbit lives with his mother and his sisters, Flopsy, Mopsy and Cottontail, in a safe burrow under a tree. Mother goes out shopping and warns her bunnies to stay in the woods and avoid the vegetable garden, since father was killed and put in a pie by the gardener, Mr McGregor. Mischievous Peter, however, slips under the garden gate to gorge on lettuce and radishes till he feels sick. Mr McGregor sees him and gives chase. In running away, Peter loses his shoes and jacket and escapes into the tool shed. Soaked from jumping into a watering can, Peter sneezes and gives his position away. Mr McGregor is tired after running after Peter and gives up. Peter is lost in the garden and tries to slip under a door in the wall, but he is too fat. He sees a mouse and, later, a cat watching some fish, and then hears Mr McGregor's hoe. He manages to dart past him and under the gate, towards home. Mr McGregor finds Peter's jacket and shoes and hangs them up for a scarecrow to scare the birds away. Peter's mother is cross about the jacket and shoes – he's lost clothes before – and she puts him to bed with camomile tea to ease his stomach pains while his sisters have bread and milk and blackberries for supper (Potter).

Excavation One – object and verb

Read the story out loud. In groups of four to five, choose one of the key sequences of the story and create a still image to which you give a caption, for example:

'Peter and family in the burrow'; 'Peter, being chased by Mr. McGregor'; 'Peter loses his clothes'; 'Peter sneezes in the tool shed'; 'Peter talking to the mouse'; 'Peter, ill in bed, drinks tea.'

Setting the compass

The title of a story often contains an entire synopsis of the story to come. What can be learned from this title? Is it a tale (or another kind of tail – signifier of the male of the species), an imaginative narrative of an event? Etymologically, the word *tale* is related to telling, a *spoken* narrative. Why is Peter a 'rabbit', but his siblings are called 'bunnies'?

In a tale, actions and events will affect the key protagonist, Peter Rabbit. Why might the protagonist have a mixed animal/human name? What does it tell us about this character?

Excavation Two – 'what's missing?' and/or 'what problem needs to be solved?'

In groups of four to five, quickly thought-shower ONE of the questions below and create a quick backstory scene with dialogue.

What's missing in the story might be Mr Rabbit – recreate the scene of his death/cooking the pie, or Mr Rabbit instilling authority in the family, or bringing home a wage to provide for food.

The problem to solve might be the idea of the Forbidden Garden. This is where Mr Rabbit came to an end and Mrs Rabbit forbids the children to go there. But the garden contains all the best food! So, the problem to solve here is, can I disobey parental authority and follow my gut (literally)? Create an alternative scene to solve this problem (e.g. purchasing vegetables from Mr McGregor or helping him with the gardening in return for food).

Excavation Three – what is naughty? Gender switch

In groups of four to five, each student selects a different dramatis personae. Students create a role on the wall from listening to the story again. Taking the characteristics of the role, students now bring the still image from the beginning of the unit to life, adding action and dialogue *but* the roles have switched gender. Peter Rabbit is now female; the sibling bunnies are male; Mr McGregor is Mrs McGregor; and so on. Devise appropriate names, keeping the concepts laid out above intact, for example, a human name for the protagonist, nonhuman names for the bunnies and so on.

Whole-class reckoning

How has the story changed, if it has? What 'male' characteristics of Peter does the audience accept that might not be so readily accepted in a female version of the story (mischievousness, nakedness, disobedience, gluttony)? How does this affect or change the relationships within the rabbit family, if at all? The naked rabbit – can a female reveal her free, natural body as Peter does? Will the male siblings still obey their mother? What do we feel about a naughty female behaving in this way as opposed to naughty Peter? What do we feel about punishment for this behaviour? Look at active and passive roles in the tale – are the sibling rabbits blob-like, flopsy, fluffy, without individual characters? When a female follows instinctual drives, do we celebrate her escape from the oppression that forces her to be passive, obedient and accepting? If we replace Peter with a female role, we maintain either/or opposites. Is there another solution?

Excavation Four – names and pronouns

Continue the idea that the protagonist in this tale might be male or female and avoid gendered language. It's useful to find a non-gendered name like PRabbit and use 'they' instead of 'he' or 'she'.

Explain the layers of the psyche:

The id (subconscious, instinctive desire) is represented by the instant pleasure-seeker PRabbit, with animalistic, needs, wants and desires. PRabbit even moves to a more animalistic form when running on four legs and shunning the jacket and shoes.

The ego (reality) might be represented by McGregor and the three bunnies at home who work conscientiously for their food and follow the rules to get their needs fulfilled.

The superego (morality) might be represented by MRabbit's super logical authority (Mrs Rabbit in the original story) warning PRabbit of the consequences of their actions, and giving out punishment, or McGregor and the pie punishment.

In groups of three, create a scene with PRabbit as protagonist and their two **alter-egos** with thought-tracking. For example, the moment PRabbit is caught in the net with alter-egos provided by M. Rabbit, McGregor, bunnies, the sparrows and so on. By the way, a small reflection on the gender of the sparrows and cat could also be enlightening!

Excavation Five – the turning point

In groups of four to five, quickly thought-shower the key turning point of the whole tale and create a still image with a caption to capture that moment.

Resetting the compass

Does the turning point resolve the problem stated at the beginning of the tale? What learning or change, if any, has the chosen character undergone?

Excavation Six - links

In the same groups, quickly thought-shower other tales that might compare. For example, Hansel and Gretel (gluttony), or tales of the youngest prince who endures obstacles before becoming a man (Sleeping Beauty), or tales of authority quashing youthful adventure (Snow White).

Create a still image of the comparison tale and practice shifting shapes from the still picture of the turning point of PRabbit just completed to the turning point of the comparison tale over a slow count of 10. Share.

In conclusion, whole-class reckoning

By reversing gender roles in this tale, the idea of two oppositional gender types – feminine and masculine – is maintained. The feminine is associated with passive, obedient, docile, seeking-to-please characteristics and the masculine with active, disobedient, risk-taking, more self-centred, ambitious characteristics. This is known as binary opposition. While changing genders in a tale may reveal prejudices and biases, it doesn't address the idea that gender could be something that exists on a wide spectrum of possibilities that is a fluid state of becoming, rather than belonging to one or other fixed and closed sense of identity entirely opposite to another kind of fixed, closed sense of identity. By taking any tale and switching the genders, students are made very aware of rigid and binary either/or approaches to gender.

Resources, Peter Rabbit

Potter, Beatrix. *The Tale of Peter Rabbit*. London: Frederick Warne, 1902; 2002.
Nodelman, Perry. "Making Boys Appear: The Masculinity of Children's Fiction." *Ways of Being Male: Representing Masculinities in Children's Literature*. Ed. John Stephens. London and New York: Routledge, 2002: 1–14.

Shifting the perspective - part 2

SITA'S RAMAYANA

The Ramayana (meaning the Journey of Rama) is an epic Sanskrit story told across India and much of East Asia that has been orally transmitted since about 7BC. It relates the story of the life of Rama, a legendary prince; Ravana, his arch enemy; Sita, his wife; and Hanuman, the Monkey King and his army, as well as thousands of other important dramatis personae along the way. Boys in India are told 'be like Rama'; girls are told 'be like Sita'. The tale is traditionally narrated from Rama's perspective – at least, he is the hero and focus of the action and drives the plot forward. However, a simple shift in perspective to Sita reveals some thought-provoking issues for drama. There are several versions of the epic with regional and cultural variations, and one of these is a Bengali version written by Chandrabati who was one of the few female re-tellers of the epic in the 16th century. Her version tells the epic from Sita's point of view:

> Rather than divide the world into good and bad, right and wrong, Sita's vision encompasses all those who suffer, endure and bear the consequences of what kings and wars do . . .

not only women children and ordinary people, but also animals, birds and nature. (Arni and Chitrakar 151)

Samhita Arni's retelling of Chandrabati's Ramayana, with Moyna Chitrakar's illustrations, using traditional Patua scroll painting techniques, is the basis of this excavation (see 'Resources, Sita's Ramayana').

Excavation One – the power of language

Narrate:

In the country of Ayodhya lives a King Dasharath with his three wives. It is a patchwork family: Dasharath has four sons: Rama, Lakshman, Shatrughna and Bharata; Bharata is the only son of one of his queens, Keikeyi. Now Dasharath feels he is too old to reign and wants to name Rama, the eldest son, his heir. Queen Keikeyi reminds Dasharath of the time she saved his life and he promised her two wishes. She commands him to banish Rama for 14 years and insists her own son, Bharata, take the throne.

Scene 1: **'As shadow to substance, so wife to husband'**

Cast: Keikeyi, Manthara and Dasharath.

Keikeyi's maid, Manthara, explains the rights of inheritance to the queen. She persuades Keikeyi to demand Bharata take the throne. Keikeyi and Manthara speak in a different language from Dasharath so when Keikeyi speaks to Dasharath there may be some interpretation/translation mistakes and/or inconsistencies. This scene must be played in different languages (made up if necessary). Reflection: who has linguistic control over the story?

Scene 2: **to obediently accept one's lifelong duty (dharma) without demur**

Cast: Dasharath, Rama, Lakshman and Sita.

King Dasharath has no choice but to fulfil his promise to Keikeyi and must banish Rama who accepts his fate. With brotherly love, Lakshman decides to follow, and, Sita, Rama's wife, is obliged to follow too (as shadow to substance, so wife to husband).

In small groups, choose ONE of the above scenes to recreate and share.

Survey the terrain 'as shadow to substance, so wife to husband'

In small groups, discuss and compare Keikeyi/Sita; Keikeyi/Dasharath; Dasharath/Rama and Rama/Sita.

Who holds the power to change events?

Excavation Two – abhinaya: guiding the performance towards the spectator

In groups of three, recreate Rama, Lakshman and Sita setting out on their exile. Break the action of travelling with each role thought-tracking in turn.

Setting the compass

What different perspectives are driven by the gender, status, dharma of each role?

In traditional Indian dance theatres, abhinaya is a technique for drawing focus onto something on stage. For example, actors use the eyes for more than just responding or looking at something. The movement of the actor's eyes as they follow a gesture can direct the spectator's attention towards an action, a place or part of the body (Coorlawala 230). It need not be the actors' eyes that draw spectator attention to something. Abhinaya can also be achieved by shifts between the narrator-third-person voice and the role-first-person voice in order to draw closer attention to the intensity of emotions. This is not unlike Brecht's Verfremdung technique where the narrator tells what the actors are doing as they do it. In this excavation, add a narrator to the stage with Rama, Lakshman and Sita, who will intercut a narrative story telling with their inner thought-tracking in order to direct the audience's eyes and ears to something of significance (spotlighting).

Think, pair, share

The technique of drawing attention to key emotions and moments through abhinaya.

Excavation Three – active versus passive

Teacher narrates: the three are tired and rest. Suddenly Sita sees a beautiful deer ahead. The arch enemy Ravana has sent a demon, disguised as a deer, to entice Sita. She begs Rama to fetch it for her. Rama reluctantly leaves Lakshman in charge and goes off to capture the deer, but it leads him deep into the forest. Suddenly, Lakshman hears Rama calling for help. He doesn't know what to do. Lakshman draws a magic circle around Sita and tells her it will protect her as long as she stays inside it. He goes off to help Rama. Sita is alone in the magic circle. Now the enemy, Ravana, tries to get Sita out of the protective circle. He may not enter the circle, nor can he touch her as long as she is inside the circle.

Mark the circle on the studio floor and have one student take up the position of Sita inside it. Students should approach, one by one, as Ravana, with, tricks, disguises, anything they can think of to get her out of the circle. Will she stay or will she leave the circle? Is her fate in her own hands?

Narrate: Ravana uses a trick to get Sita under his control. He dresses as a beggar needing help. Of course, she comes out of the circle to give him food. She is caught, kidnapped and taken to his kingdom, but when she refuses to be Ravana's wife, she is imprisoned. Sita sits in prison, guarded by rakshasas and rakshasis. Choral speech: the rakshasas and rakshasis are cruel and taunting, singing Ravana's praises as a great leader, and trying to persuade Sita to give up Rama and marry Ravana to save herself. Ravana thinks time will change Sita's mind.

Survey the terrain

How is this confinement different from the confinement of the magic circle?

Narrate:

Meanwhile Rama and Lakshman have returned and, seeing the empty circle, raise help from Hanuman and the army of monkeys. There is a terrible battle of destruction leading, finally, to victory for Rama and Hanuman. Hanuman destroys the palace and gardens with fire, 'It was as if time had stopped flowing'. Everything has been decimated. Ravana is killed.

Whole-class improvisation

Read the passage below, narrated by Sita.

Fruits and leaves rained down. Creepers and branches were trampled into the earth . . . and on and on . . . ravaging the beautiful gardens in flames, smoke filled the air, children coughed, lungs filled with soot and dust . . . I heard the women of the palace, shrieking. I saw Ravana's queens running to the battlefield, tears streaming down their faces. Their screams rent the air. Even I, enclosed in this garden, could hear their grief. They would be queens no more, and their people had met death on the battlefield – for what? For one man's unlawful desire. Men had been killed, women widowed, and children orphaned. It was such a high price to pay. . . . (Arni and Chitrakar)

Students recreate the soundscape that Sita hears alone, locked in her prison, as she waits for Rama to come and rescue her.

Whole-class reckoning

In small groups, discuss the power of 'passive' non-action.

Excavation Four – rasa: showing emotions

Narrate: silence falls. Time passes. Rama does not come for Sita for a long time because he's 'busy'. Finally, Rama does not come for Sita himself but sends Hanuman instead. Hanuman brings Sita to see Rama:

RAMA: (aloof, distant, angry) Sita you are free. I have freed you. You can do whatever you want. Go wherever you want.

SITA: What did he mean? I was stunned.

RAMA: Ravana must have touched you. I can't have you back.

SITA: Why did you fight this war? If you said you weren't coming, I would have killed myself.

RAMA: I fought the war for my honour, not for you.

SITA: So many people are dead; women and children are lost; the battlefield is drenched with blood and corpses. I thought the end of the war meant freedom for me. I had hoped for love. I had hoped for justice. That was not to be. Instead of love I found suspicion. Instead of justice I met with false accusation and distrust. (Arni and Chitrakar 115-119)

In traditional Indian dance theatre, emotions only 'happen' when they land in the minds and hearts of the audience. The emotions are not simply 'mixed by performers and handed to the audience on a platter' (Schechner 107). In this tradition, all the performance and production elements come together in the spectator's mind/gut/eyes/ears. The term 'rasa' is used to describe this 'gut emotion or feeling' that is stirred in the spectator. It can sometimes be translated as 'flavour' or 'taste', like a meal made up of mixtures of sweet, sour, bitter and spicy elements.

Rasa graffiti

There are eight basic 'flavours' of rasa emotion, plus shanta, which is 'nothingness' (see Table 2.1).

Table 2.1 Eight 'flavours' of rasa emotion

Rage	Disgust	Fear, shame
Pity, grief	Shanta (nothingness)	Desire, love
Humour, laughter	Energy	Surprise

Divide the studio floor into nine boxes with chalk or tape.

Allocate the eight rasa emotion flavours to different boxes. The order does not matter, except shanta, which must remain in the centre. Shanta can be a resting place, a neutral place.

Ask students to reflect in silence on experiences, responses, moments associated with at least five of these rasa flavours. Students should write these on sticky notes and attach them to the appropriate box. During this exercise, do not allow the students to enter the boxes. They should remain on the lines between or outside the grid before moving to each box.

Once everyone has finished, allow students time to read the stickies on each box and reflect in silence. No need to explain or question.

Students choose one of the rasa flavours and explore a physicalization of it, remembering facial expression, body tension, centre of gravity, levels, closed/open, soft/hard and so on. There is no need to think deeply, seek truth or originality. The goal is to explore the difference between experiencing an emotion and expressing it outwardly. Once the still image of one rasa is fixed, choose two more and repeat.

Move between the chosen rasa still images by jumping or walking along the lines of the grid. Explore the rapid shift between rasas – there is no slow transition or development, simply an automatic, muscle memory response as students land in the different boxes and transform into each rasa emotion flavour. The aim is to work from an outer, objective physicalization (Chapter 3 on mask in this book may also help) to an inner, subjective feeling that communicates outwardly to the spectator.

Explore vocalization sounds such as laughter, sighs, phrases or words that belong to each of the chosen three rasa flavours.

In pairs, with both actors on the grid and using the dialogue of Rama and Sita above with pauses, repetitions and silences, explore how the dialogue changes by simply moving between the prepared three rasa flavours.

Setting the compass

Inner feelings and outward show – is there a gender difference?

Excavation Five – leaders and followers

Narrate: Sita takes the honourable solution and offers herself up for sacrifice by allowing herself to be burnt on the pyre in the traditional way for widows. But the fire does not touch or harm her, and she steps from it unscathed, proving her purity. Rama accepts her back and Rama, Sita and Lakshman arrive back in Ayodhya. Their return is marked by Diwali, festival of light. (Art classes may consider making clay Diwali lamps and drawing mandalas to recreate the celebrations.) But Rama is troubled about taking Sita back and believes she has been unfaithful to him, so he sends her away.

Solo mime: students choose to represent either Sita, sitting at the edge of the water considering what to do or, Rama having sent Sita away, in a still image. Remind students to consider body tension, centre of gravity, levels, facial expression and so on. Once the image is fixed, ask all those playing Rama to sit. All the Sitas take up their position over a count of 10, before slowly sinking to a sitting position at the teacher's command. Then all those playing Rama should slowly rise into their positions over a count of 10.

Survey the terrain

Similarities/differences in the physicality of Sita and Rama. In the opening scenes, Sita was 'As shadow to substance, so wife to husband' – has Sita's role changed? Has Rama's role changed? What do the still images show?

Excavation Six – not either/or, but also

Traditional Indian dance theatre shifts between narration and enactment, between third person narrative and first-person speech, gesture and action. Spectators are constantly being asked to accept the theatricality of the performance (recognize the people on stage are just acting) and at the same time be moved by the actions, gestures and speech of the characters to an emotional response. In this way, there is no one single way of watching or interpreting what's happening on stage – the spectator has to manage identifying with the emotions and characters as well as staying at a critical distance. This double effect, or dual focus, being both 'in' and 'out' of the story occurs through the explicit oppositions within the story: good/bad; dominant/subordinate; masculine/feminine. These opposites give the spectator a choice between good/bad, real/false, masculine/feminine that keeps shifting. A single, firm view of things is not an option (Nair 239).

Students find a partner who has chosen a different role from their own in the last excavation. Teach each other the still image. Review the story from the beginning, marking notable moments, actions, phrases or words for each role. Add these to create a duo physicalization by layering, combining, fusing and/or shifting between the representation of the two roles, Rama and Sita. Share this double-body performance.

In conclusion, whole-class reckoning

The position of power or dominance need not automatically fall to a masculine role.

By position of power, we might mean the power to change events, power to take action, power to change minds, power to have control over one's own journey. Can anyone claim that power?

Resources, Sita's Ramayana

Arni, Samhita and Moyna Chitrakar. *Sita's Ramayana*. Chennai: Tara Books, 2018.

Coorlawala, Uttara Asha. "An Alternative to Male Gaze." *The Natyasastra and the Body in Performance. Essays on Indian Theories of Dance and Drama*. Ed. Sreenath Nair. Jefferson, NC: McFarland and Company, 2015. 229–245.

Nair, Sreenath. *The Natyasastra and the Body in Performance. Essays on Indian Theories of Dance Drama*. Jefferson, NC: McFarland and Company, 2015.

Schechner, Richard. "Rasaesthetics." *The Drama Review* 45.3 (2001): 27–50.

Shapeshifters (growing sideways) – part 1

Allerleirauh - Bristlehide

Stories that contain shapeshifters, transformers, humans and animals and/or humans and machines present an alternative to the idea that one is *either* this *or* that. It presents a model of *both* this *and* that and thus neatly introduces the idea that gender might be something marked along a spectrum and that gender might also change over time, many times and in time. Gender can be a fluid, changing concept. Kathryn Bond Stockton suggested a new term for the evolution of identity as '*sideways* growth', to replace the concept of growing *up* on one predetermined track, signposted by elders and fixed. In sideways growth, the development can take different turns off a particular track; one is free to collect experiences rather than give up one identity for another (Fairfield). It suggests a process of becoming – of trying on different physical shapes or shapeshifting. The students will know a wide range of stories in videogames, books, television and film that might fit into this genre. Have them make a list!

Bristlehide synopsis

Grimm's tale Allerleirauh (All-kinds-of-fur), which I have translated as Bristlehide, can be found as number 65 in the original version of the Tales of the Brothers Grimm from 1812. This is a synopsis and not the original, which should ideally be used instead (Zipes). As the king's wife lies dying, she asks him to remarry but only if he can find another as beautiful as she, with the same golden hair as herself. The king searches across the kingdom but cannot find anyone as beautiful. One day, he sees his own daughter and decides she is the spitting image of his deceased wife and he will marry her. The princess is horrified and sets him three tasks as a condition of marrying that she hopes are impossible to fulfil: he should make her a dress as golden as the sun, a dress as silver as the moon and a dress that sparkles like the stars. She also demands a cloak made of a thousand different animal furs and that a piece of skin from every species of animal in the entire kingdom should be attached to it. With the help of all the young women weaving and hunters hunting, the king succeeds in all the tasks and provides the gifts. So, the princess makes a bundle of these items and three charms given to her by her true fiancé, the prince: a golden ring, spinning wheel and bobbin and puts them into a nutshell. She clothes herself in the animal hair and skin cloak, blackens her face and hands with soot and escapes into the forest in a faraway land. She finds a hollow in the base of a tree to sleep. Her fiancé and his men are hunting nearby and discover a wild animal never seen before. They catch it, tie it up and bring it to work in the kitchens doing all the low and menial tasks. In the evenings, the wild animal has to pull off the prince's boots for him and he always throws them at its head afterward, so it isn't a pleasant job. The wild animal lives in a dark hollow under the stairs. One evening, a ball is planned, and the wild animal sneaks away to wash and dress, transforming itself into the princess again, wearing the golden dress. Of course, the prince falls in love with her when they dance, but she runs away, resumes the bristlehide cloak and returns to the kitchen. There, the wild animal makes the prince some soup and drops the ring from the nutshell in it. When the prince drinks the soup, he is amazed and calls for the cook. The cook says it was the wild animal that made the soup. The wild animal is called for and says it has no idea how the ring came into the soup. Another ball is arranged, and this time, the wild animal changes into the silver moon dress and dances with the prince. On its return the wild animal slips the spinning wheel into the soup and the same thing happens again. The prince is frustrated. At the third ball, he arranges for the music to play longer than usual, so that the princess in the starry dress is kept dancing. He forces a ring on her finger and tries to stop her from running away. But she escapes. Back in the kitchen, the wild animal does not have enough time to wash properly, so when the prince comes down to the kitchen, he notices poking out of the cloak a white finger with his ring on it. He tears off the cloak from the wild animal and the starry dress shows through and the princess's golden locks appear. He realizes it is his fiancée, the beautiful princess, and they marry and live happily ever after.

'Allerleirauh', the name of the wild animal, contains the word for 'all kinds of' (all kinds of being). The term rauh means rough, rude, uncultured, native, hairy, gruff, bristly. The story models ambiguous bodies: the princess who is the spitting image of her mother with golden hair, and the wild animal that is untamed, bristly, whiskery, dirty, dishevelled, rough and raw, dirty, crude and rude. In the original German, the narration slips in and out of personal pronouns: 'she', 'her' for the princess and 'it', 'it's' for the wild animal – an appealing structure to explore what it means to be golden-haired 'feminine' or 'wild/dirty/rough/hairy 'masculine'. Moreover, the three magic dresses of sun, moon and stars are just as much a disguise as the bristlehide rags of the rough cloak, so there are several 'guises' at work here.

Excavation One – masculine/feminine

Read the story aloud.

Students should write down all the signs in the story they associate with 'femininity': queen, princess, golden hair, beauty, spinning wheel, spindle, cooking, cleaning, sewing the three dresses, the three dresses, white skin and so on.

Now they should do the same for 'masculinity' or 'not-feminine': black face, bristlehide, cloak, soot, hovel, hunters, king, prince, boots, wild and so on.

In groups of four, plot these gender ideas in the story on a Venn diagram (see Figure 2.1).

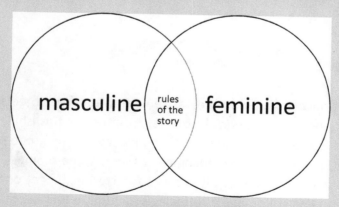

Figure 2.1 Story gender.

A second Venn diagram (Figure 2.2) should now be filled with so-called 'feminine' and 'masculine' objects and activities and so on in the real world as we experience it today.

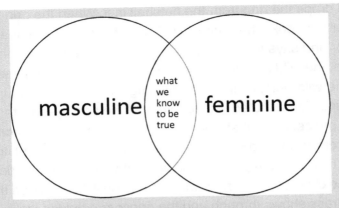

Figure 2.2 What we know to be true.

Does this diagram look like Figure 2.3? If it doesn't, why not?

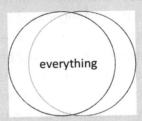

Figure 2.3 Ideal gender diagram.

In groups of four, choose mantle of the expert role play to investigate the bristlehide cloak that was recently discovered by archaeologists in your area:

As archaeologists discovering and questioning the find

As historians and cultural researchers preparing materials to put the cloak on display in the local museum

As newspaper reporters preparing a piece on the find for the local evening news

Share the reports in role

Survey the terrain

What are the 'signs' of masculine and feminine, if any: objects, appearance, dress, jobs?

Excavation Two – metamorphosis

Students create the princess's room in the castle with a few real objects left behind before the escape. All actors on stage represent objects, furniture or furnishings in the room. One student, as king, enters the room and discovers she has gone. The group secretly whisper the princess's secrets, hopes and fears as the king passes around the room.

Without further discussion, instruct all actors to move in silence, one by one, to centre stage to build a whole-class still image of the king's nightmare fear for his daughter.

Setting the compass

Small group discussion: the environment reflects inner desires.

Excavation Three – language

In groups of five to six, recreate the campfire. The hunters in the forest have captured bristlehide and are chatting about the wild animal. What are they thinking? How do they talk about it? What kind of vocabulary do they use? Why? Share.

Excavation Four – shapeshifting

Divide the class in half.

Group A work in pairs: student X moulds student Y into the realistic external shape or pose of the princess. Once the figure is fixed and X is satisfied, Y now moulds X into the spiritual shape of the princess.

All group A onstage with all Ys as realistically outwardly presented princess and spiritual inner soul Xs behind them. Ys slowly sink to the floor to reveal X, the inner selves, the different inside images of the role. Share with group B.

Group B work in pairs: the same exercise above with the realistic and inner shapes of Bristlehide. Share with group A.

Whole-class reckoning

Does the outside reflect what's inside?

Excavation Five – inside out and outside in

Introduce the terms:

Assigned sex: the gender given by the medical profession at birth by looking at the baby's genitalia. However, bodies come in many forms and lots of people don't fit this mould.

Gender: 'the state of being a man, a woman, both, neither, somewhere in between or something entirely different' (Mardell 61).

Binary: either/or – society dictates that there are only two gender categories, and everyone belongs to only one or the other.

Gender expression: a person's own sense of their gender. It can include clothing, language, body language, name, appearance, but it can also be private. Gender expression can also be changeable from minute to minute, month to month or year to year, that is, gender fluid. Gender scientists write about 'becoming' rather than 'being'. Nothing is fixed.

This is theatre, so we are discussing role, not sexual attraction such as homo-, hetero- or bisexuality. Make a clear distinction, since one's gender expression is not automatically linked to the person to whom one is sexually attracted.

Gender expression or identity can be expressed as a spectrum (Figure 2.4) rather than a binary system of opposites, either/or.

masculine ⟵——————————————⟶ feminine

Figure 2.4 Gender as spectrum.

Run through some of the key characters in the story and ask students to stand on the spectrum at the point they believe these roles in the story lie: the king, the queen, the princess, the prince, the hunters and so on. Where would bristlehide stand? Why?

Excavation Six – disguise

Create a scene - In groups of four, design a piece of clothing for a current-day version of the character bristlehide/princess to escape in. Create a workshop scene with actors sewing, gluing, cutting, chopping, welding, baking to demonstrate what it's made of, how it was made and why these choices were made. What items from today's world would contribute to the clothing and why? Choose a name for the character (Allerleirauh means all kinds of bristly fur or hide) that derives from the materials used in making the disguise. Share and follow with class discussion.

Excavation Seven – the reveal

At the end of the story, when the prince comes down to the kitchen, he notices the wild animal's white finger with his ring on it. He tears off the cloak from the wild animal and the starry dress shows through and her golden hair falls down. He realizes it is his fiancée, the beautiful princess.

Explain that a famous sculptor has created a statue of the moment of revelation. Working in pairs, have student A model student B into the sculptor's statue. All the Bs should present the statues while all the As walk around them to observe and comment to each other.

Whole-class reckoning

The ending of the story – which statue seems most believable? Why? Does the story provide the kind of resolution that the princess was seeking when she escaped her father? Can the statue capture all aspects of the princess's nature in the story? Is it important to capture them? How does the prince 'see' the princess now?

Excavation Eight – it's in the bag

In pairs, create a scene:

Two good friends sit together chatting about school life. A plastic bag lies on stage with an unknown disguise (clothing, props) inside. Is the disguise still in use? Will the audience know it is a disguise? Will the audience learn what the disguise consists of or will it all remain secret? Where is the plastic bag during the conversation? Do the friends talk about it? Do both know what it is (explore the subtext)? What happens at the end of the conversation? Will the disguise be thrown away? Opened? Prepare and share.

In conclusion, whole-class reckoning

What disguises do we use in everyday life? For what purpose? Disguise or revelation?

Resources, Bristlehide

Fairfield, Joy Brooke. "Becoming Mouse, Becoming Man. The Sideways Growth of Princess Mouseskin." *Transgressive Tales: Queering the Grimms*. Eds. Kay Turner et al. Detroit, MI: Wayne State University Press, 2012. 223ff.

Mardell, Ashley. *The ABCs of LGBTQ+*. Coral Gables, FL: Mango Media, 2016.

Zipes, Jack. *Don't Bet on the Prince. Contemporary Feminist Fairy Tales in North America and England.* New York: Routledge, 2012.

Zipes, Jack (Ed.) "All Fur." *The Complete First Edition of the Original Folk and Fairy Tales of the Brothers Grimm*. Princeton, NJ and Oxford: Princeton University Press, 2014. 216–220.

Shapeshifters (growing sideways) – part 2

OVID'S METAMORPHOSES

'Of bodies changed to other shapes I sing' (Ovid). The world of Greek mythology is inhabited by an array of humans who are either punished for wrongdoing and transformed into animals and objects (trees, flowers, stones) or who choose those forms having suffered unbearable violence and pain or who seek transformation as an escape to freedom. The transformed figure sometimes loses the power of spoken language and is unable to communicate. Sometimes this is an advantage and relief. Sometimes other aspects of the transformation enable flight or much-needed strength. The transformed figure frequently loses the power of movement and becomes fixed or frozen. Yet, it still lives and sees and feels and experiences life from the outside, not unlike the Invisible Boy in Chapter 3.

Excavation One – the resource

Below are listed some of the transformative dramatis personae from Ovid's Metamorphoses:

Actaeon changed into a stag
Aesacus changed into a diving bird
Aglauros changed to dark stone
Alcyone changed into a kingfisher
Arachne changed into a spider
Arne Sithonis changed into a jackdaw
Attis changed to a pine tree
Cadmus changed into a snake
Callisto changed into a bear and into a constellation
Cycnus turned into a swan
Cyparissus changed into a cypress tree

Daedalion changed into a hawk
Echo changed into just a voice with no body
Hecuba changed into a dog
Hermaphroditus merges with Salmacis to form one person
Hyacinthus changed into a flower
Iphis changed from a girl into a man
Lycaon turned into a wolf
Medusa's hair changed into snakes
Mestra changed into a fisherman
Midas was given asses' ears
Myrrha changed into a tree
Narcissus changed into a flower
Nyctimene changed into an owl
Ocyrhoë changed into a horse
Orion's daughters' ashes changed into two young men
Perdix changed into a partridge
Philomela changed into a nightingale
Procne changed into a swallow
Pygmalion's statue changed into a living girl
Salmacis merges into one person with Hermaphroditus
Smilax changed into bindweed
Teiresias changed to a woman and then back to a man
Tereus changed into a hoopoe bird. (I. Johnstone)

Choose a shapeshifter that inspires you and research all you can about them. The stories are often quite short, so you may have to do some imaginative work to fill in the blanks.

Second, do some research about the object of transformation, its qualities, appearance and specifics. You may like to find images as well to get a sense of the shape, size, texture, colours. Put the two pieces of research together, as shown in Table 2.2.

Table 2.2 Shapeshifter research organizer

Lycaon	King of Arcadia	Barbaric, but also cultured	Name means 'she-wolf' and 'of the light'	Think they're better than Zeus	Had 50 sons
Wolf	Territorial, dominates their domain	Pack hunter preying on the vulnerable; feeds first before feeding pups; devours internal organs first; sociable, runs in packs	Howls to mark territory, no connection to moon phases; Greeks associated wolf with Apollo, God of Light and Order	Natural enemies are rare – occasionally bear, tiger, lynx, but these are fights over food	Wolves live in packs of up to 40 or so

Excavation Two – physicalize

From your transformation story, identify the moment of change and highlight any key words to help you find physicalizations for the before and after of your chosen character.

Working individually, find the physical body shape of your chosen dramatis personae. What stance, body tension, centre of gravity, or facial expression best catches this person? Once a shape has been found, starting from a neutral stance, move to the stance over the count of 10, pacing the movements to finish exactly on the last count. Then reverse the movement back into neutral over the count of 10.

Now find a body shape for the transformed figure/object. What shape, body tension, centre of gravity, facial expression are needed to catch its essence? Once a shape has been found, starting from a neutral stance, move to the transformed stance over the count of 10, pacing the movements to finish exactly on the last count. Then reverse the movement back into neutral over the count of 10.

Choose which of the rehearsed forms to begin with and adopt this stance. Over the count of 10, slowly transform into the second shape; pause for 3 long seconds.

Whole-class reckoning

Can a different physical shape of the body change the mind? What happens if the transformation is reversed back to the original?

Excavation Three – internalize

Return to the research of your story and select five significant words or create some words and phrases of your own from the tale. Play with your physical transformation deciding which words to speak and when and how to speak them during the transformation process.

Thought-shower a sound that might ease the physical transformation and explore how to add it to the moment of transformation. In film, sound provides continuity between shots allowing for coherence. The sound you choose may be a sound effect, a typical sound from the environment or actual animal sound of your figure. You may prefer a small piece of music but do not use music that has lyrics. Rehearse, refine, share.

In conclusion, whole-class reckoning

How does the outside world see/hear the body's inside? In Philip Pullman's *His Dark Materials*, Lyra has a daemon or animal spirit. If you had an animal spirit, what animal would it be and why? Lyra's daemon changes form several times. Why might this be? Compare the different effects of transformation imposed by others or chosen by self.

Resources, Metamorphoses

Hughes, Ted. *Tales from Ovid*. London: Faber and Faber, 2009.

Johnstone, Ian. "Ovid Metamorphoses." 2017. *johnstoniatexts.x10host.com*. Professor Ian Johnstone. 24 March 2020. <http://johnstoniatexts.x10host.com/ovid/ovidtofc.html>.

Ovid. "Ovid's Metamorphoses, tr. Anthony S. Kline." 2000. *The Ovid Collection*. 24 March 2020. <https://ovid.lib.virginia.edu/trans/Ovhome.htm>.

Being invisible

Postcards from No Man's Land

The title of the novel, *Postcards from No Man's Land* (Chambers), is the starting point for a piece of collaborative devised theatre. The novel describes 17-year-old Jacob's journey to Amsterdam to learn about his grandfather's death in World War II but in doing so he discovers much more about himself. He sends postcards home documenting his journey. It is difficult to de-gender *No Man's Land*. 'Man' technically refers to all humankind, but it should be explained from the start that in this unit *No Man's Land* can simply mean 'the place in between' as it was used in the *Doomsday* book to describe the land between two fields, 'belonging to no one'.

Excavation One – rules of engagement

In groups of four to five, start some quick research about the definitions and kinds of No Man's Land that exist(ed) in the world and in time. These might include examples such as World War I, the Iron Curtain, the Bamboo Curtain, the Cactus Curtain and so on.

Discover and discuss: what's inside, what's outside? What obstacles make the land difficult to transverse? What debris scars the land? Who controls No Man's Land? What are the boundaries of No Man's Land? What are the rules of No Man's Land? Unoccupied? Under dispute? Entrenchment? Sense of displacement and not belonging?

Download the pamphlet, 'This is not an Atlas' (This is not an Atlas) that explains how to create 'counter' cartographies, or maps of the world that do not map geographies. Perhaps there are some ideas here for you to develop a Counter Cartography for your No Man's Land.

Excavation Two – the ally

Taking the answers to these and other questions the group may have about real situations of No Man's Land around the world, choose a fictive situation where No Man's Land might be interpreted metaphorically as a place of in-between. Choose a protagonist who will be sending the postcards and a distant recipient/ally who will be receiving them. Name both characters and build an identity for each (role on the wall/building a character).

Ally: 'a member of the majority or dominant group who works to end oppression by recognizing their own privilege and supporting or advocating for the oppressed population' (GLSEN).

Excavation Three - postcards

Create a series of five postcards (still images) of the situation over a period of time as it changes for the protagonist and ally.

Create a caption for each of the postcards and find a way to include this in the still images.

Excavation Four - writing

Create a message written by the protagonist to the ally/recipient and find a way to communicate this in/through/above/over the still images.

Excavation Five - responding

Create a way to include responses by the ally/recipient of the postcard. Find moments where the focus shifts from protagonist to ally/recipient to show two sides of the story.

In conclusion, whole-class reckoning

Displacement: how was the feeling of 'not belonging' presented in the pieces?
   Vacancy: how was the feeling of being neither/nor presented in the pieces?
   How is the role of ally significant in the pieces presented?
   Must No Man's Land be a negative experience?
   Other thoughts?

Resources, Postcards from No Man's Land

Chambers, Aidan. *Postcards from No Man's Land*. Definitions, 2007.
GLSEN. *GLSEN.org*. 2019. March 2020. <https://www.glsen.org/>.
"This is not an Atlas." n.d. *This Is not an Atlas.org*. Kollektiv Orangotango+. March 2020. <https://notanatlas.org/book/>.

Breaking out - mirrors windows doors

KAFKA'S *BEFORE THE LAW*

The Secret Garden, Alice in Wonderland, The Lion, the Witch and the Wardrobe, Coraline, are but a few of the many examples of Anglo-American children's literature premised on the concept of transition or portals between worlds: a door, a wardrobe, a mirror, a tunnel, a window. The access to the other world is often dangerous, limited in time and open to certain 'qualified' individuals only, but passage changes the individual forever.

Excavation One – mapping

In groups of four to five, students thought-shower some favourite examples of doors, windows and mirrors that act as portals in literature, film, videogames. Share and discuss.

Before the Law was first published in 1919, a decade after its author, Franz Kafka, graduated in Legal Studies from the University of Prague. Kafka was a German speaker from an Ashkenazi Jewish family living in predominantly Czech-speaking Prague. His work is permeated by a sense of alienation and feeling trapped in an incomprehensible and maze-like world of foreign-dominated administration and authority. He felt ostracized by everyone since he did not belong to any community, religion, society, language or culture around him. There are countless academic studies of this tale for further research if desired. Judith Butler derived her concept of 'performing gender' from Jacques Derrida's interpretation of this story, 'the one who waits for the law, sits before the door of the law, attributes a certain force to the law for which one waits . . . I wondered whether we do not labor under a similar expectation concerning gender' (Butler xv). Sociocultural 'rules' of gender seem to prevent a broader, more fluid understanding of gender expression and identity. There is no final truth, or 'there' behind the door, but there is a momentary truth in the 'here' and 'now'.

Synopsis

The tale itself is short enough to read in full. However, Theodore Ushev has created a haunting animation of it (available online) – 'The Man Who Waited' (Ushev) – which will serve as starting point for this section. It was reportedly the first film made specifically for the cellphone in 2006. The tale was not intended for young readers and is agonizingly open-ended. But it is precisely this open ending (open beginning and open middle) that challenges the reader/audience to work to create meaning and allows for any meaning and every meaning. A man 'of the earth', a simple person, comes to a door, which is open. In front of the door stands a doorkeeper. The man asks the doorkeeper if he may pass through the door and access the truth/the law within. 'It is not possible, for the time being', says the doorkeeper. 'And tomorrow?' he asks. 'Not yet' is the reply. The door to the truth/the law is always open but, since he cannot enter, the man waits by the door. He waits days; years. He is near death. Before he dies, he asks, 'If everyone is searching for the truth, why am I the only one who has asked to enter?' The door keeper replies, 'This entrance is yours alone. No one else may enter here'. The door closes.

Excavation Two – listening

Each student sits alone with paper/whiteboard and pens. Play Ushev's video with sound only and ask students to write and draw what they hear, see, feel, taste, touch in the telling of the story. Repeat once more with visual only. Find a partner, share and discuss.

Excavation Three – opposition and ambiguity

Staying in these pairs, students now watch the film complete with images and sound. On second watching, ask students to document as many pairs as they can: sits/stands; mind/sight; maybe/not yet; and so on. Explain the difference between oppositions in a *dialectic* discussion, where two viewpoints are stated, then move towards resolution and compromise and *dialogical* discussion where conflicting positions are unresolved, left hanging, ambiguous, but in relation to one another. Dialogic means related to everything that ever has been and ever will be said. So, in this sense, the pairs found by the students are not necessarily complementary or oppositional; they are left 'hanging', in the air, unresolved and unexplained.

Survey the terrain

What possible meanings are implied by this story? Being cowed by authority? Senselessness of authority? Faceless authority? Everyone is equal before the truth/law? What significance is there in that both doorkeeper and man are outside the door? Who or what is Inside and who or what is Outside? Who 'belongs'? Who has control? What web of concepts can be spun that this tale helps to reveal?

Excavation Four – to act or not to act?

In pairs, find another pair to make a group of four and discuss the story and its lack of resolution. Students should quickly jot down questions that the story raises, for example: what is the protagonist seeking? Why does the protagonist stop seeking? Is it wrong to stop seeking? Why has the protagonist been denied access to the truth? What power is it that holds 'the truth' and refuses to share?

In these groups of four, review notes, sketches and ideas and agree on an interpretation. Prepare a short piece for presentation that must include:

- A set comprised of one table and two chairs (these are the only props used in traditional Chinese theatre. They can represent a mountain, a bed, a military camp, a bridge or a table and two chairs). There must be at least two set changes.
- A soundtrack (not music), either live or recorded, to create atmosphere and/or environment.

Setting the compass

The individual searches for what? Obstacles faced in the search? Individual responsibility to act or to not act.

In conclusion, whole-class reckoning

Underpinning Shakespeare's Hamlet is the question 'to be or not to be'. Hamlet battles with conflict between being and doing, which has always been interpreted as a negative thought process that destroys his mind and ultimately leads to his tragedy. However, could the idea of non-action allow for 'everything to be possible'? Could the ambiguity of non-action actually offer a kind of freedom?

Resources, Before the Law

Butler, Judith. *Gender Trouble*. New York and London: Routledge, 1990.
Ushev, Theodore. "The Man Who Waited." 2017. *Facebook.com.* March 2020. <https://www.facebook.com/theodore.ushev/videos/1861440944100247/>.

Integration of identity (for now) – part 1

Just a regular Joey

The search for identity is often described as a journey out, a journey away from family, friends, even country – from everything that is known and familiar. Freud spoke of the integration of the three parts of the mind – the id, ego and superego – and only when all three were finally united in one body could one say a person was whole. In literal terms, the traveller has had to learn to integrate all new experiences, self-discoveries and emotions into a new understanding of self. Finally, weary, but changed, the traveller returns home. How will they be accepted and integrated into society again? This section is based on a picture book, *Normal Norman* (Perceval). A small child is perfectly happy until suddenly waking up one day with a pair of wings. The child tries to hide the wings from everyone by putting on a bright yellow coat to cover them, but the coat is hot in summer, and inconvenient at bath time. In the end, the child takes off the coat and discovers the joy of using the wings and flying. While flying, the child realizes other children and adults around also have wings.

Excavation One – just a regular Joey

Class discussion

What is 'normal'? What makes a 'normal' teenager? Is it appearance? What is the 'normal' of fashion now? What kind of slang is 'normal'? What kind of music is 'normal'? What do teenagers 'normally' do after school? What kind of behaviour is 'normal'?

   In groups of five to six, create a role on the wall for Joey. Followed by whole-class discussion.

Excavation Two – what does normal look like?

Introduce character: Joey (regular kind of student) averagely popular, averagely good looking, averagely intelligent. Keep gender flexible – and use 'they' as a pronoun rather than 'he' or 'she'.

   In groups of four to five, create a scene with the sort of 'normal' actions and dialogues that happen among young people among friends: lunch in the school cafeteria; bus ride; at the ice cream parlour; sports team practice; choir practice; and so on. Joey can be included in these scenes. Spotlight the scenes randomly around the room, by starting and stopping back and forth between group pieces to catch the language style and content of typical teenager talk.

Excavation Three - Joey at home

Solo mime: Joey at home. Dim the studio lights and have students close their eyes, each working in a small, defined area. Narrate Joey returning home after school one day, exhausted. Flings the schoolbag onto the floor and collapses onto the bed. Thoughts of the day run through Joey's head. As Joey, students should model where and how Joey sits/lies/stands in the bedroom. Students formulate three key thoughts of Joey and repeat these in their head. Ask students to speak the thoughts aloud. Find different intonations for these thoughts. Mulling, playing with volume, tone, timbre.

Excavation Four - Joey changes

Solo mime (continued)

Narrate that Joey eventually drops off to sleep. Teacher-in-role calls, 'Joey! Joey! Wake up, dinner's ready!' Narrate that Joey wakes and feels a bit weird, different somehow. Joey reaches back and discovers a pair of wings sprouting from the shoulder blades. Joey is horrified/amused/ delighted/puzzled. What does Joey feel about this new body? Give students time to run through some thoughts in their head. Teacher-in-role calls, 'Joey! Joey! Wake up, dinner's ready!'

Excavation Five - disguise

Solo mime (continued)

Narrate that Joey realizes it's time to go down to dinner. What to do about the wings? Joey decides to hide them by using some kind of disguise. How will this be done? With a hoody/ thick jumper/jacket/coat? What is Joey thinking at the top of the stairs before going down to dinner? Students create an inner thought, then speak it out loud along with the whole class in an increasingly chaotic cacophony of words, getting louder at each round: whisper it, speak it, speak it louder, shout it, then whisper again and turn the door handle to go down to dinner.

Extension

Improvisation with teacher-in-role as parent, playing devil's advocate by standing at the bottom of the stairs looking up at each Joey in turn - urging, demanding, persuading, mocking, begging them to 'cover up' or 'take off' the disguise and come down to dinner. Will any student come down?

Think, pair, share

How was Joey feeling before/after discovering the wings? Did Joey decide to hide the wings or not? Obviously, the wings are a metaphor for something Joey wants to hide from others. What do you think the metaphor is? What is Joey really trying to hide? Why does Joey feel it has to be hidden? Discuss.

Excavation Six – reactions

Whole group recreates a street scene with one student, randomly selected, or teacher-in-role as Joey. The ensemble creates a street scene. Each group decides on specific kinds of people one might meet on the street – all ages, all types, pairs, groups, single. Make the street scene as realistic as possible, people moving, people stopping, small actions and so on. Once the scene is rehearsed and fixed, Joey enters. Joey walks to catch the bus to school next day. Still wearing the disguise. How do the people on the street react to Joey in the disguise?

Setting the compass

What is normal? Is it normal to look away? Is it normal to feel not normal?

Excavation Seven – the expert

Small groups create the roles of Joey, a doctor, parent(s)/guardian(s). The scene is set in hospital where Joey has been brought to discover if there is any medical/psychological solution to the 'problem'. Start the scene with parents/guardians and Joey waiting for doctor. Spotlight various groups before allowing the doctors in each group to enter and continue the scene in any way they choose.

  Charting the terrain: what's Joey going to do?

Excavation Eight - forum discussion

Two lines of chairs facing each other. Divide the students randomly.
  Line A thinks Joey should take the disguise off and see what the wings can do.
  Line B thinks that Joey should continue to keep the wings a secret.
  One student from each line begins the discussion by standing. If a student runs out of arguments, anyone in their line can whisper another argument to the student standing. If the student has truly run out of arguments, they can sit down, and another student can stand and continue. But each student can only stand up to argue once. At the same time, teacher steps er to one or other line to show which 'side' currently seems to be 'winning'.

sion, whole-class reckoning - where next?

ce showing Joey removing the disguise (could be real, could be a dream).
piece showing Joey and all the others removing their disguises.
7 at a social event.
ey – aged 43 in role, what happened to Joey as adult? Take one aspect from
a group piece.

Choral speech – to sum up Joey's feelings at a chosen moment, or (as Greek chorus) to comment on a dialogue happening between Joey and one other character from the story.

A devised monologue for Joey or one of the characters in the story.

A soundscape for the moment of disguise or reveal.

Resource, Just a Regular Joey

Perceval, Tom. *Normal Norman*. London: Bloomsbury Books, 2017.

Integration of identity (for now) - part 2

The queen bee

The protagonist in this story is Simpleton, a frequent figure in the Grimm stories (Zipes 208–210). Simpleton is usually the youngest of three brothers, whether princes or paupers, someone everyone thinks is foolish and no one takes seriously (in a man's world). However, through his natural charm, he is able to harness magical powers that transform him into a mature adult who wins the day. Features that make this character stand out are the inability to 'learn' the rules of society; he is not a rebel, he just doesn't care; and he behaves in a way nobody in society would expect or understand. He is a kind of outsider. Sometimes Simpleton is said to have 'feminine' qualities as he is uneducated (as many females of the day were). He is a dreamer, since he has empathy with nature and a spontaneous generosity. A name switch to 'Innocent', rather than 'Simpleton', shows the parallel well. Simpleton seems to lack 'masculine' qualities such as logic, muscle and bluff. Simpleton represents the instinctive, natural, subconscious world or acting without thinking. Simpleton's communication with creatures is a common motif in such stories – appearing in Snow White and Cinderella as positive expressions of being in touch with natural and inner expression. In this tale, Simpleton makes a journey that develops understanding of his identity as a mature person.

Synopsis

Two princes go out looking for an adventure and lose their bearings, following a wild, decadent way of life, which means they can't find their way home. Simpleton decides to go out and look for them. He finds them, but they mock him for thinking that he could make his way in the world as he is such a fool, when they, who were much cleverer than he, had failed. They travel together for a while and come upon an anthill. The older brothers want to smash it for fun and watch the ants crawl away in fright, but Simpleton says, 'Leave the little creatures in peace, I can't bear to let you disturb them'. Next they come to a lake with many ducks. The brothers want to catch some to roast and eat, but Simpleton says, 'Leave the creatures in peace. I can't bear to let you kill them'. Finally, they arrive at a beehive and the brothers want to set fire to the tree where it hangs, so as to get to the honey, but Simpleton says, 'Leave the creatures in peace. I can't bear to let you burn them'. Finally, the brothers arrive at a deserted castle. Inside is a door with three locks. In the middle of the door is a peephole through which they spy a little grey man. After the third time of calling he comes out to them, invites them in to eat and drink and shows them to their rooms. The next day, the little man shows the oldest brother a stone tablet engraved with three tasks. If anyone can perform all three tasks, the castle will be released from its enchantment. Task one is to gather 1,000 pearls belonging to the king's daughter scattered in the moss throughout the forest. If, by sundown, one single pearl is missing, the seeker will be turned to stone. The oldest brother only finds 100 pearls and is turned to stone. The second brother tries, but he only finds 200 pearls and he too is turned to stone. Simpleton tries his luck, but quickly fails and begins to weep. The ants whose lives he had saved come by and quickly gather up all the pearls for him. The second task is to fetch the key to the princess's room from the bottom of the lake. At the lake, the ducks whose lives Simpleton had saved, dive down to bring the key to him. The third, and hardest task, is to pick which is the youngest and loveliest of the three princesses. They all look the same. Before dropping off to sleep, each has eaten a different sweet: the oldest ate sugar, the second ate syrup and the youngest ate honey. The Queen Bee, whose life Simpleton had saved, comes by and tests the lips of the princesses. She recognizes the honey on the lips of the youngest princess and the spell is broken. All the sleeping forms inside the castle that were once stone now come back to life. Simpleton marries the youngest daughter; his brothers marry the 'less beautiful' sisters.

Excavation One – outside looking in

The way everyone else sees Simpleton

In groups of four to five, create small scenes demonstrating the kinds of foolish things Simpleton does as illustrations for a story book. Provide a title for the illustration, 'Simpleton . . .' Share.

The way everyone sees the brothers

A large group of 12 peers are sitting with their phones, chatting on social media about the behaviour of the two older brothers who are 'out in the world' and 'behaving badly'. Speak the texted, tweeted, Instagram messages and images as they come in. Using gossip, jargon, hashtag, likes, shock, mock condemnation or admiration, share-with and so on to provide a soundscape of media words and phrases to describe the brothers. Share.

The way Simpleton sees himself

In pairs, thought-shower what objects and things Simpleton would take on his journey and why he would take them. One student sits in the centre as Simpleton with an imagined or real suitcase. Students approach and put the objects into the suitcase, gifting him as they explain how it will be useful to him. At the end, Simpleton may choose only three and explain the choice.

Survey the terrain

What is missing? Why does Simpleton go out on the journey? What is he really looking for?

Excavation Two – whole-class-forum challenge

Review the concept of a whole, or integrated identity having three levels: the id (pleasure-seeking, instinctive, desiring, inherited, aggressive, drive by urges) located in the subconscious, the ego (observes rules taught by the external world, makes decisions, follows social etiquette, can rationally devise a method of achieving a goal but does not care about right or wrong too much) and the superego (the authority figure, the adult, the moral viewpoint set by a culture that controls impulse, knowing how to treat others and what it feels like to do wrong).

In small groups, students should quickly thought-shower to identify specific characters in the story in terms of id, ego and superego, for example:

Older brothers representing the id, driven by desires.

Simpleton representing the id, transitioning to ego transitioning to superego in forbidding the slaughter.

The ants, ducks and bees representing the superego, rational authority.

What do the princesses represent?

In pairs, pick out the various motifs and unpick their potential meanings in the tale. For example:

Ants – earth, hard-working, providers, nurturing community, cooperation.

Ducks – water, dark depths, diving to the depths of the soul.

Bees – air, produce honey from nectar, transformative, cycle of life, the Queen Bee as the ruler of the hive.

Castle – a symbol of the self with all its closed doors and stone, dead statues.

Pearls – the most beautiful treasures are hidden under the forest floor – in order to find them, one needs to be in touch with nature and the emotions.

The key at the bottom of the lake – the key to the princess's inner self, the key to one's feminine nature.

Sugar and syrup – fabricated processed sweetness, produced by slaves.

Honey – natural sweetness, pollination, cycle of life, sting, serving the community.

Class chooses one of the scenes: ants, ducks or bees. Arrange chairs in two lines facing each other. One line will be filled with students playing Simpleton arguing to save the creatures; the opposite chairs are filled by those playing the older brothers who want to destroy them. At any one time, there can only be one student from each side arguing their case. Once a student has run out of arguments, another member of the team can whisper an idea. Alternatively, the student sits and another member of the same team tags in. Each student can only stand and speak one time. At the same time, the teacher can move between the two lines to show, by their position, which line is 'winning' the argument at any one time.

Excavation Three – two worlds

Solo reflection

The castle might represent the sleepy self, the unconscious; it has many doors and corridors and windows, but all are locked, and the inhabitants are turned to stone. What might be behind those doors?

Whole-class improvise

Create still images of the spirits locked inside the doors of the castle. Have them come to life very slowly, speaking their feelings and thoughts as they do so. A cacophony of waking up.

Class discussion

What world had they fallen asleep in and what world have they woken up in?

Excavation Four – the space between

What became of the brothers and their wives? Did they change their ways? Did they start to appreciate and understand Simpleton? Model the space between Simpleton and his brothers at the beginning of the story showing how close or far their relations are to each other (proxemics). A different group of students now model the space between them.

Survey the terrain

Has the relationship in the family changed? Why? Why not?

Excavation Five – flashforward

In small groups of four to five, create a scene showing who Simpleton becomes, what kind of person, at any age of your choosing. Make sure the scene includes an action by Simpleton that reflects his state of id, ego or superego.

In conclusion, whole-class reckoning

Identity, and the exploration of self, is a lifelong journey and that's OK.

To what extent might identity be shaped by intellectual, physical, familial, religious, sexual, educational, gender, peer, racial and/or cultural influences and who has control over these?

Resource, Queen Bee

Zipes, Jack (Ed.) *The Complete First Edition: The Original Folk and Fairy Tales of the Brothers Grimm*. Princeton, NJ and Oxford: Princeton University Press, 2014. 208–210.

Recognition of 'other'

Dare to be different

A role model is not necessarily a mould that everyone must fit into. It can also simply be a model of different possibilities for consideration and understanding. The more we encounter different models or ideas of the world, the better the understanding we will have of our own position. Two books will provide the material for this section: *Stories for Kids Who Dare to Be Different* (Brooks) and *Queer, There and Everywhere – 23 People Who Changed the World* (Prager), but you probably have your own heroes too. Both books provide real-life examples of both famous and less famous people who have 'invented, radicalized and trailblazed'; who have defied gender limitations and/or found a way to be themselves. Also included in the resources are two books containing personal accounts from young people today.

The Theatre of the Oppressed created by Augusto Boal is a perfect tool to explore real lives in theatre, particularly, Newspaper Theatre. Boal said, 'We think theatre should be a game the whole world can play . . . You do not need to be a speaker to participate in a meeting, you do not need to be an athlete to play football' (Boal). Boal's Newspaper Theatre was aimed at exposing the manipulation of information in mass media and offering a contrasting perspective to get at the truth. His theory is driven by political objectives on matters that affect a local situation where the theatre is being created and the need to challenge and awaken a desire for change.

Excavation One – who?

In groups of four to five, browse the suggested biographies and narratives in the resources and agree a key protagonist upon whom to base a performance piece. Discover all you can about your chosen person. Find different kinds of text about them, not just Wikipedia. Look for video interviews, social media, reviews of their work; look for examples of the work they have done; photos of them and their backgrounds, families, activities, culture.

Excavation Two – for whom?

Prepare a performance piece on your chosen figure that will challenge, surprise, enlighten and inform the spectators. You can include banners, projections, voiceovers, as well as live performance. Be very clear before you begin what your objective is in telling this story. What do you want the spectators to take away with them? What are your intentions in shaping the story?

Excavation Three – how?

Look at Table 2.3 Newspaper Theatre Techniques. Find a way to combine, include, cut into, fade into, crossfade, juxtapose, swipe, project, some techniques to really give your material and message a punch!

Table 2.3 Boal's newspaper theatre techniques (Boal 234)

Simple reading	Read a text about your figure as a report, word for word
Complementary reading	Read as a report but add information that might be missing but still important, that the original report deliberately omitted

(*Continued*)

Table 2.3 Continued

Cross-reading	Choose two reports from entirely different sources that show two different perspectives on the story to demonstrate that information is manipulated
Remove adjectives	Remove all descriptive words from the text to get to its essentials
Rhythmical reading	For example, read the text to the rhythm of a rap, a march, a tango to create different associations with the text. This will emphasize different aspects of the story
Reinforced reading	Add extra content in between the texts such as advertisements, breaking news, political or cultural events that might be relevant to the texts or that help to give context to the text
Parallel action	A group acts out its version of the story while it is read by another. The actors need to make anything that is hidden in the spoken version as explicit as possible
Abstraction	Create a gap between the content of the text and what the speaker is doing; for example, the reader might be putting up shelves or ironing, while the reading is about impending nuclear war
Social media readings	Include tweets, texts, 'likes' hashtags and so on that challenge or reinforce chosen aspects of the story
Historical reading	Connect the text to other texts that connect to relevant moments in another time period
Global reading	Connect the text to other texts that connect to relevant moments in another part of the world
Improvisation	Improvise the scene that the story describes
Text out of context	Change the context of the news story being presented
Insert into actual context	For example, in a text dealing with gender-based violence, add other texts that might demonstrate similar oppressions
Redefinition	Stop the text at any point to explain any euphemisms, unclear or derogatory vocabulary, explaining what the problem with the vocabulary is
Empathy	Add information that explains the feelings of some characters in the text. This may not be written down anywhere, so you may have to invent some

In conclusion, whole-class reckoning

What themes or ideas have emerged from these performances? How does Newspaper Theatre compare with, say a biopic at the movies, or a more naturalistic enactment of moments of a person's life?

In your groups, discuss any changes you would like to make to the person's life to give it a perfect happy-ever-after moment if it doesn't have one. How would this change affect the telling of your story?

Resources, Recognition of 'Other'

Boal, Augusto. *The Routledge Companion to Theatre of the Oppressed.* Eds. Julian Boal and José Soeiro Kelly Howe. London: Routledge, 2019.

—. *Legislative Theatre.* London: Routledge, 2005.

Brooks, Ben. *Stories for Kids Who Dare to Be Different.* London: Quercus, 2018.

Finney Boylan, Jennifer. *Stuck in the Middle with You. A Memoir of Parenting in Three Genders.* New York: Crown Publishers, 2013.

Gold, Mitchell, ed. *Crisis. 40 Stories Revealing the Personal, Social and Religious Pain and Trauma of Growing up Gay in America.* Austin, TX: Green Leaf Press, 2008.

Prager, Sarah. *Queer, There and Everywhere. 23 People Who Changed the World.* New York: Harper, 2017.

And finally . . .

This chapter has introduced a small selection of potential children's literature that may serve as starting points for your drama class. As you look for your own examples, bear these criteria in mind that were suggested by the Council on Interracial Books for Children when they expanded their mission to include sexism:

1. Check the illustrations or avoid illustrations. (Bettelheim suggested that illustrations detract from the learning process rather than foster it, because the illustrations direct the child's imagination away from how they, on their own, would experience the story; Bettelheim 60)
2. Look for tokenism – what roles are allocated gender types; are both genders active or inactive; are they leaders or are they subservient?
3. Plot: does the story require a stereotypical solution – a girl has to behave like a boy in order to succeed? Is the child who does the most understanding and forgiving a girl, and is the child who resolves the problem a male?
4. Whose interest does the hero serve?
5. Does the story ask a character to strive to be normal in a way that would limit their view of themselves? Is the story open to anyone and everyone?
6. Review the author's biography to consider perspective and bias.
7. Consider any loaded vocabulary and look out for sexist language; look out for use of terms such as ancestor, not forefather; firefighter, not fireman; community, not brotherhood; manufactured, not manmade.
8. Check the date of writing – a few non-gendered children's books started to appear in the 1970s, but since the 2000s there is better understanding of the issues and representation of gender.

Resource, *Critical Multicultural Analysis of Children's Literature*

Botelho, Maria Jose and Masha Kabakow Rudman. *Critical Multicultural Analysis of Children's Literature.* New York: Routledge, 2009.

CHAPTER 3
Without gender - mask

Master Wang Yuechun had a round, moon-shaped face. He was chosen for the painted-face role because of it. His head was completely shaved, as were his brows. He wore a wide, cream-coloured cotton shirt, tied diagonally at one shoulder, and baggy blue regulation trousers, wrapped and also tied at the side, with regulation black, cotton-padded shoes. Master Wang was going to teach me how to paint my face. Every painted-face character in traditional Chinese theatre has its own fixed pattern. The colours and symbols of each face tell the audience a story about the character: white for deception; red for loyalty; a bat for good fortune to the actor's performance; an axe to show the killing done by the character in the coming story. These face patterns have stayed the same for hundreds of years and cannot be changed. Each one is instantly recognized, just as Red Riding Hood's costume tells us who she is, so do the individual face patterns of the generals tell the audience precisely which character stands before them on stage.

First, I copied onto paper in pencil the face of Zhang Fei, a cheery, friendly general. I marked the blocked areas and noted the lines dissecting the face from nostril to chin, from inner eye to cheekbone. I added a character description, with arrows pointing to the patterns on his face that give this away. Because my face is not round or moon-shaped, Master Wang gave me a piece of silk to tie over my forehead and over the hairline in order to extend the size of my paintable area. The white powder and water mix covers the face first. Then, using black ink and water (the same ink used in calligraphy: it stains!) I marked out the three key areas of the face and the lines that would transect it. The brush is soft and thick – if you press hard, it makes a thick mark; if you press lightly, a thin one. You have to hold it like a calligraphy brush at 90 degrees to the face so you can start a thicker line and sweep across the face as it thins to a point at one end. Your face is full of valleys and hills, unlike paper, but you can manipulate the brush against these mountainous formations to create exquisite darts and sweeping waves. Once the pattern is set in black ink and Master Zhang has approved, you can start to add the oily white base between the black markings and then the oily reds, blacks and pinks, filling in, shaping, shifting the facial structure through colour-blocking and lines that draw the eye of the spectator. The face begins to glisten with the oil; it's hot on your face, even though the classroom temperature in winter in Beijing is the opposite, icy cold. The mirror gives back my imperfect reproduction, but I cannot think it is me. I am lost in this new apparition – the cheeks are broad, the forehead wide, the eyes

DOI: 10.4324/9781003080800-4

fiercely covered in black to the nostrils, the mouth downturned and lipless. I feel so different. I do not look like me. I am not me. Master Wang's expertly painted face at the opposite end of the room is striking. He tilts his face, angles it, to catch the light or shade, opens his eyes wider than wide, moves his mouth, blows out his cheeks, raises an eyebrow, frowns, then stretches his mouth. The character he is representing comes alive. The face is distorted and different in perspective. It isn't Master Wang. It's a face full of wild expressiveness, more than human, artificial.

He nods at me, back in himself again. Not satisfied with my efforts, he commands me to wash it all off. The water gushes out of the taps in freezing bursts. The primitive soap barely cuts through the oil on my face, thick as car lacquer, and I leave class with raw, red, very sore cheeks, marked by black stains and a memory of a transformation so great I am still breathless.

Mask demands letting go of one's own identity and expressing another. Mask can avoid discussion of gender altogether; at the same time as it can challenge gender stereotypes by using comedy.

In 1872, Charles Darwin claimed that facial expressions of emotion are 'universal, not learned differently in each culture; they are biologically determined, the product of evolution' (Darwin). More recent scientific research suggests that the statement is largely true. There are some slight cultural differences, but there is very little difference between people of different race, gender or age, in the way the face expresses emotion (Ekman 23). The human face may be described as having a universal language of performance. Exploring mask work is the perfect dramatic form for understanding and playing with identity that is free from gender signs or boundaries. This first section will focus on the full mask covering the entire face; the second section explores the painted face of Chinese traditional theatre; and the third section will focus on the half mask of Italian Commedia dell'arte.

The face

Edward Gordon Craig was happy to dispense with human faces in theatre altogether:

> What I tell is not new; it is what all artists know.
> Human facial expression is for the most part worthless, and the study of my art tells me that it is better, provided it is not dull, that instead of six hundred expressions, but six expressions shall appear on the face of the performer. (Craig on Theatre 20)

The actor's biologically given face, and the use of a mask to disguise, distort, or elevate it to represent another, is fundamental to performance across the world in time and space. In ancient Greek theatre, an actor was called 'hypokrites' (two-faced), because they wore masks on stage, suggesting a clear divide between the actor as 'being' and the actor as 'representing' another being, not themselves.

Barely a culture in the world has not created mask for ritual, ceremony and/or performance including: the theatre of the ancient Greeks; mystery plays of the Middle Ages; European exorcist rituals at New Year; Chinese Nuo exorcist theatre; Japanese No theatre; Roman 'persona' masks; Japanese Kyogen theatre; 17th-century English masque; Italian Commedia dell'arte; 18th-century harlequinades; sacred Lhamo dramas of Tibet; Topeng of Bali; ritual and ceremonial masks of the Yoruba; Igbo and Edo cultures and Egungun masquerades of sub-Saharan Africa; Maori masks of New Zealand; woven masks of the Caribbean; neutral and larval masks of Jacques Lecoq; Talchum in Korea; Brazilian and Caribbean carnival; Melanesian ancestor worship masks; masks among the Inuit, North American Hopi, Navaho, Zuni and Iroquois masks; and many more. Craig continues:

> Drama, which is not trivial, takes us *beyond reality* and yet asks a human face, the realest of things, to express all that. It is unfair. . . . Masks carry conviction when he who creates them is an artist, for the artist limits the statements which he places upon these masks. The face of the actor carries no such conviction; it is over-full of fleeting expression – frail, restless, disturbed and disturbing. (Craig on Theatre 21)

Craig is determined to rid the stage of human beings altogether since the expressions they produce are too unstable, too changeable, '. . . the body of man . . . is by nature *utterly useless* as a material for an art' (Craig on Theatre 83). Instead, he envisions artworks created by artists that will replace human failings, since:

> Art arrives only by design. Therefore, in order to make any work of art it is clear we may only work in those materials with which we can calculate. Man is not one of these materials. . . . The actions of the actor's body, the expression of his face, the sounds of his voice, all are at the mercy of the winds of his emotions and these winds. . . . As with his movement, so is it with the expression of his face. The mind struggling and succeeding for a moment, in moving the eyes, or the muscles of the face whither it will; the mind bringing the face for a few moments into thorough subjection, is suddenly swept aside by the emotion which has grown hot through action of the mind . . . with the actor, emotion *possesses* him; it seizes upon his limbs, moving them whither it will. He is at its beck and call. (Craig, On the Art of the Theatre 82–83)

Faced with a clear division between the 'real/biological' face and an 'artificial/art-mask' created by an artist to communicate directly and cleanly, the task of the actor is to explore ways to animate, breathe life into and make the art mask 'come alive'.

Mask design, or score

Craig mentions six expressions fundamental to the actor's skill. Curiously, nearly a century later, psychologist and pioneer in the study of facial expression and emotion, Paul Ekman, also identified six basic emotions shared and understood universally by most cultures:

> Surprise, Fear, Disgust, Angry, Happy, Sad. (Ekman)

However, Ekman did notice slight differences between cultures since people had been taught to manage or control their facial expression or emotions in specific culturally determined situations. In his book, *Unmasking the Face*, Ekman defines two areas of the human face used to express emotion: the forehead, the eyebrows and eyes all working as one; the cheeks, nose and the mouth as another. Ekman details how different emotions are composed of these elements and their interaction. In this book, I will use the term 'score', like a musical score, for describing a theatre system that documents several lines of different facial 'instruments' that come into play together to create one sound, like an orchestra. It is a term I will use throughout this book, borrowed from Robert Lepage, who uses 'score' to document all the performance and production elements that work together in layers within one moment of one performance. Ekman himself compares facial expression to a system of road signs where the shape of a road sign (triangle, square, circle), its colour (red, blue, green), and any words, drawings, and numbers on it, all transmit different messages in combination about rules, warnings and information (Ekman 10).

The design of a mask, therefore, needs to respect the score, or layers of meaning if it is to be 'believable'. Craig suggests capturing the 'essence' of an emotion in the mask. The drawing of a donkey with the words 'this is a donkey' underneath it is superfluous. A child can already see that it's a donkey, so the mask artist needs to create the impression of a donkey, the spirit of the thing, so that it doesn't have to be named. Ekman's book is extremely helpful in defining how to 'read' basic emotional clues or 'essences' of emotion. In each case below, the first example shows both sections of the face, upper and lower, expressing one emotion. Mixed emotions are created when the top or bottom half of the face expresses a different emotion, for example: 'questioning surprise, dumbfounded surprise, dazed surprise, slight, moderate and extreme surprise' (Ekman 1). Use your hand to cover the upper and lower halves of the face to see how the different facial elements combine. These drawings provide useful templates for creating nuanced masks of emotion which can then be used in the following excavations.

Surprise (Figure 3.1)

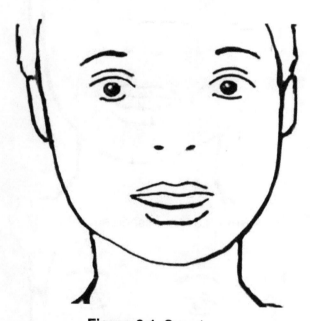

Figure 3.1 Surprise.

The brows are raised so they are curved and high. The skin below the brows is stretched. Horizontal wrinkles go across the forehead. The eyelids are opened, the upper lids are raised, and the lower lids drawn down, the whites of the eyes show. The jaw drops open so that lips and teeth are parted, but there is no tension or stretching of the mouth (Ekman 45). Surprise can have a range of 'mixed' emotions as well. See Figure 3.2, questioning surprise; Figure 3.3, astonished surprise; and Figure 3.4, dazed surprise. Put your hand over half the face to see the two different emotions in one face.

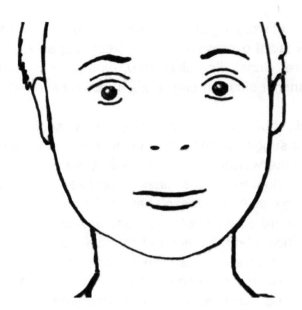

Figure 3.2 Questioning surprise.

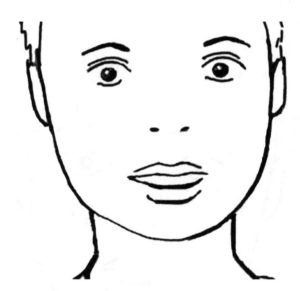

Figure 3.3 Astonished surprise.

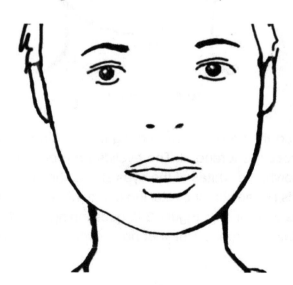

Figure 3.4 Dazed surprise.

Fear (Figure 3.5)

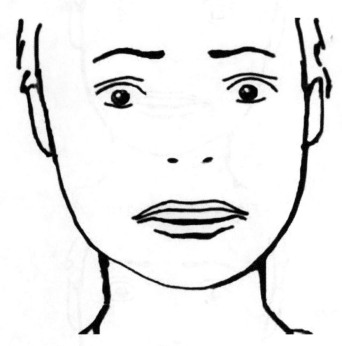

Figure 3.5 Fear.

The brows are raised and drawn together. Wrinkles in the forehead are in the centre rather than across the entire forehead. The upper eyelids are raised, exposing the whites, and the lower eyelids are tensed and drawn up. The mouth is open, and the lips are either tensed slightly and drawn back or stretched and drawn back (Ekman 63). Fear can have a range of 'mixed' emotions as well. See Figure 3.6, apprehensive fear; Figure 3.7, horrified fear; and Figure 3.8, fear and surprise. Put your hand over half the face to see the two different emotions in one face.

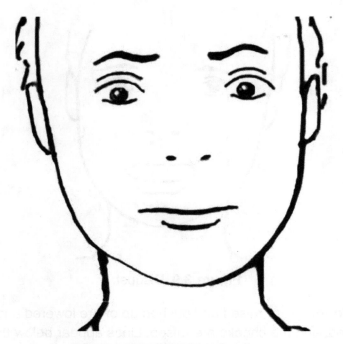

Figure 3.6 Apprehensive fear.

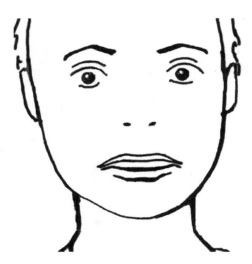

Figure 3.7 Horrified fear.

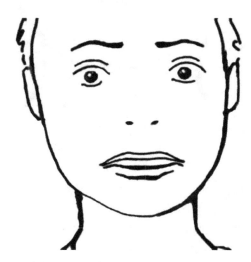

Figure 3.8 Fear and surprise.

Disgust (Figure 3.9)

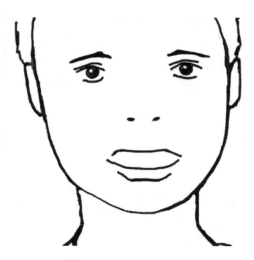

Figure 3.9 Disgust.

The upper lip and lower lip are raised and pushed up or are lowered and slightly protruding. The nose is wrinkled, and the cheeks are raised. Lines appear below the lower lids, and the upper lip is pushed up but not tense. The brows are lowered, which lowers the upper eyelids.

Disgust can have a range of 'mixed' emotions as well. See Figure 3.10, disgust and fear; Figure 3.11, disgust and disbelief; and Figure 3.12, disgust and surprise. Put your hand over half the face to see the two different emotions in one face.

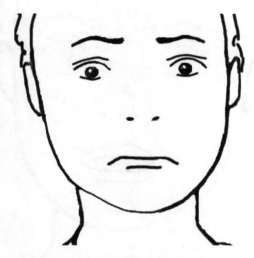

Figure 3.10 Disgust and fear.

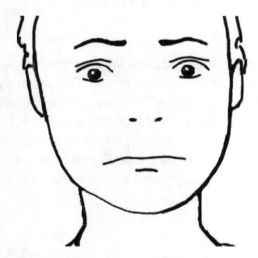

Figure 3.11 Disgust and disbelief.

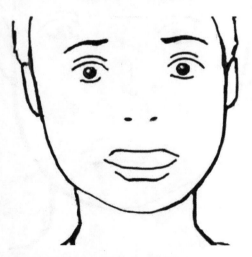

Figure 3.12 Disgust and surprise.

Angry (Figure 3.13)

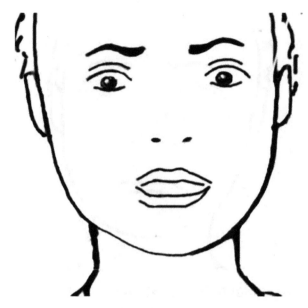

Figure 3.13 Anger.

The brows are low and drawn together, and vertical lines appear between the brows. The lower eyelids are tensed and may or may not be raised. The upper eyelids are tense and may or may not be lowered by the action of the brow. The eyes have a hard stare and may have a bulging appearance. The lips are either pressed firmly together with the corners turned straight down or open, or tensed, in squarish shape as if shouting. The nostrils may be dilated (Ekman 95). Angry can have a range of 'mixed' emotions as well. See Figure 3.14, angry and disgust; Figure 3.15, angry and contempt; and Figure 3.16, angry and surprise. Put your hand over half the face to see the two different emotions in one face.

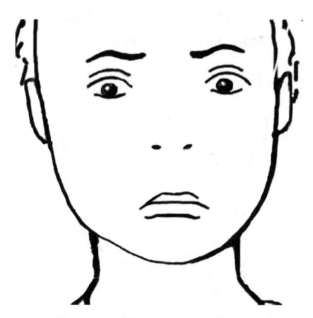

Figure 3.14 Anger and disgust.

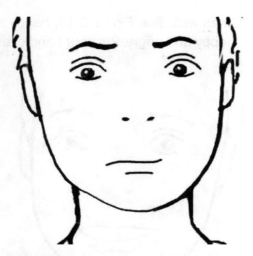

Figure 3.15 Anger and contempt.

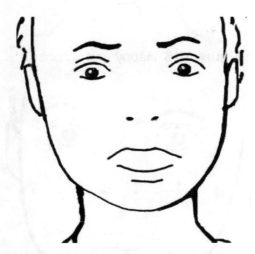

Figure 3.16 Anger and surprise.

Happy (Figure 3.17)

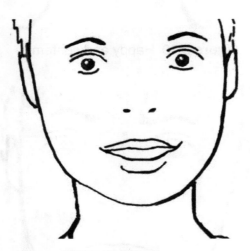

Figure 3.17 Happy.

The corners of the lips are drawn back and up while the lips may or may not be parted, with teeth exposed or not. A wrinkle appears between nostril and outer edges of the lips, and the cheeks are raised. The lower eyelids have wrinkles below them and may be raised but not tense. Crows-feet wrinkles extend from the outer corners of the eye (Ekman 112). Happy can have a range of 'mixed' emotions as well. See Figure 3.18, happy surprise; Figure 3.19, happy and contempt; and Figure 3.20, happy and angry. Put your hand over half the face to see the two different emotions in one face.

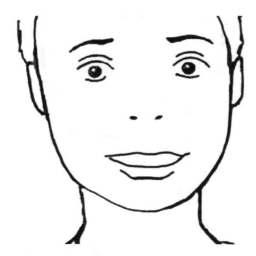

Figure 3.18 Happy and surprise.

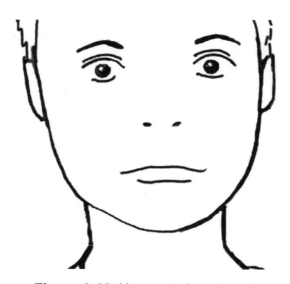

Figure 3.19 Happy and contempt.

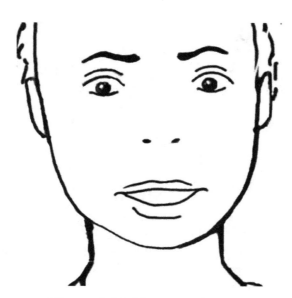

Figure 3.20 Happy and anger.

Sad (Figure 3.21)

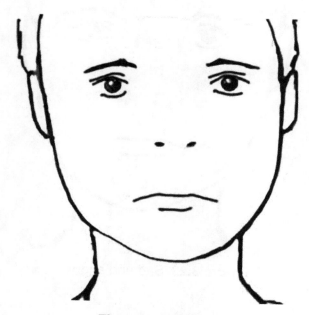

Figure 3.21 Sad.

The inner corners of the eyebrows are drawn up, and the skin below the eyebrows is triangulated, with the inner corner turned up. The upper eyelid corners are raised, and the corners of the lips are down or trembling (Ekman 126). Sadness can have a range of 'mixed' emotions as well. See Figure 3.22, sad and fear; Figure 3.23, sad and angry; and Figure 3.24, sad and disgusted. Put your hand over half the face to see the two different emotions in one face.

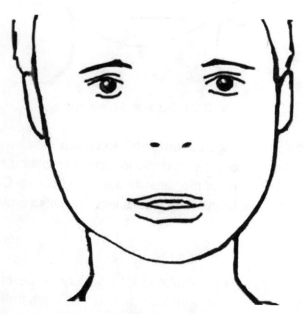

Figure 3.22 Sad and fear.

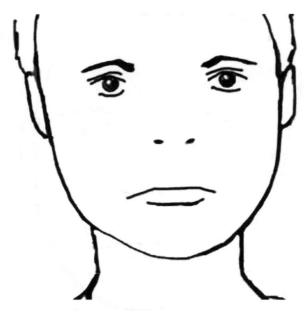

Figure 3.23 Sad and angry.

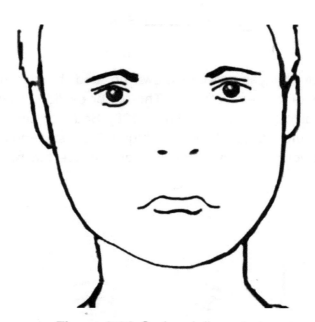

Figure 3.24 Sad and disgusted.

Students should use these drawings as templates to create their own masks. Using firm card in any colour, and black marker, encourage students to design emotions according to the direction, flow and angle of lines in both sections of the 'face' as described above. Changing the mask size to be either much larger or much smaller than the actor's face, can also prove highly effective.

Control and deceit

Facial expressions of emotion can be manipulated for a variety of reasons. There are social rules about what you are permitted to show on your face and cultural rules that tell you how to appear in public as well as rules deriving from personal habits, tics or even jobs. We are taught as children to disguise our emotions: 'don't make that face'; 'smile for Aunty'; 'boys don't cry'. The spectator has the job of deciding whether the emotions being displayed by the actor's face are 'true' or 'false'; whether the masked performance is authentic, 'believable' or not. Ex-FBI agent Navarro has some insights on reading true and false signals in the face based on whether or not the whole body is showing signs of 'comfort' or 'discomfort'. He shows how trying to disguise emotions makes people tense with 'tight jaw muscles, flaring nostrils, squinting eyes and quivering lips or biting lips, neck is stiff, no head tilt' (Navarro 167). In contrast, uncontrolled (natural) emotions are more relaxed (Navarro 169–170). The only way to perform a convincing mask is through practice, audience feedback and more practice.

Duration of emotions

The contradictory nature of mask work is that the basic expressions of emotion in the face in real life are extremely fleeting. Some facial expressions last barely a fraction of a second, and few last longer than 5 seconds, although a mood might last a longer period. However, the mask is inscribed with one, apparently fixed, emotion.

Technique: tilting

Each theatre mask, no matter from what genre or part of the world it derives, is a fixed expression of an emotion, instantly recognizable or readable by the spectator through universal facial contractions and positionings as demonstrated by Ekman. How then, can an actor make this static face come alive on stage? In Japanese No theatre, tilting the mask affects its impact on the spectator;

> when a character is sad or deep in thought, the dancer leans forward, shifting the angle of the mask more acutely downward. The change in expression is called clouding (kumorashi). The opposite effect, brightening, (terashi) is achieved by pulling the body back so the mask tilts upwards. In this position the mask seems to express a happy state of mind. (Brazell and Bethe 136)

The Trestle Theatre Mask company call this technique 'counter-mask'.

Technique: getting into mask

In many cultures, there is a ceremony or ritual to be observed before putting on the mask. In Chinese Nuo theatre, the eyes and mouth of the mask are first daubed with the blood of a cockerel

Excavation One – getting to know you

Students lie on their backs with feet flat on the floor and knees raised with eyes closed.
Align and straighten the spine against the floor.
Place hands over the lower belly and feel the belly rise as the breath is taken in and sink as breath is expired.
Let your thoughts go and focus on the steady rise and fall of the belly.
A mask will be placed on your chest, facing up, chin to chin.
Slowly open your eyes and look down at the mask.
Holding the mask at the side edges only, move the mask and your own head so that the mask looks up at you.
Peers down at you.
Looks at you from the left.
Looks at you from the right.
Notice the play of light and shadow across the features of the mask.
Lie back down, placing the mask back on your chest (Simon, Masking 32).

in a ritual ceremony to 'open' the mask to the spirit being represented (Riley 113–115). The actors fast and pray for days before the performance, first emptying themselves of their identity before putting on the identity of the mask once it has been 'opened'. Bethe and Brazell describe a similar process of respect for the mask-as-face in Japanese No theatre:

> On the day of the performance cords are slipped through the holes at the side of the mask and the mask is laid on a pillow . . . in the room adjoining the bridge to the stage. After his costume is on, and before donning the mask, the dancer holds it with both hands, then lifts it in homage. Next, he places it in front of his face, throws the cords over his shoulders and allows the stage attendants to tie the cords tightly. (Brazell and Bethe 138)

In exploring the mask, avoid the mirror or camera altogether at first. In performance, allow the audience response to guide you about whether or not your mask is believable. Listen to the audience response, react to the audience response. The believability of the mask is a collaborative agreement made between actor and spectator.

Excavation Two – mask and spectator

Exercise: less is more

1. Enter silently in mask.
2. Stand in mask facing the audience.
3. Do as little as possible as you experience being quiet.
4. Connect with your audience by looking out at them for at least 1 minute.
5. Silently accept any audience response you get – laughter, giggles, sighs, applause.
6. Exit silently in mask.

Exercise: clouding (kumorashi) and brightening (terashi)

1. Enter in mask.
2. Stand and look at the audience.
3. Practice looking at each person in the audience.
4. Keep the mask straight as you connect with the audience.
5. After a long while, slowly tilt your mask in a downward motion (clouding).
6. After a long while, slowly tilt your mask in an upward motion (brightening).
7. Choose the best of the three masks you have shown; the one that seemed to get the most reaction from the audience.
8. Exit with the chosen face, facing front, slowly (Simon, Clowning 13-16).

Excavation Three – mask as body

Put on the mask and explore a physical stance, a physicality, by standing still in a pose that captures the mask on the face through the entire body. Use the entire body focusing on body tension, centre of gravity, level, head position and tilt, shoulders, gesture, hands, hips, legs, feet. Exaggerate the pose from a 6 to an 8 to a 10. Create two more stances or typical gestures for the same mask and repeat the exercise.

   Share: in groups of three, run through each of the three stances at the teacher's call. Face front at all times. Once all three have been shown, teacher calls numbers randomly. Snap between poses quickly. Feel the audience response and make adjustments to the stance if needed.

Survey the terrain

Review the table of techniques and obstacles presented in Table 3.1 and discuss.

Table 3.1 Mask techniques and obstacles

Technique	Obstacle
Disguise the edges Make sure that hair or a hat, scarf or bonnet covers the edge of the mask, where it meets the face, to hide the deceit	Vision In Japanese No theatre, the mask has very small eyes providing extremely limited vision. Actors use the pillars at the four corners of the stage and shifts in light to judge their position on stage (Brazell and Bethe 139). What signposts can you use?
Facing the front Make sure the mask faces the front as much as possible to avoid showing the edges of the mask in profile. The face has the features that the audience needs to see to read the action and emotion	Breath The full mask does not always allow for easy breathing. The performance must be structured to provide for the actor to leave the stage and catch their breath
Proportion Exploring the size of the mask in relation to the rest of the body. However, the eyeline of the mask and the eyeline of the actor must match, so padding must be used to ensure this	Touch Any attempt by the actor to touch the mask during performance breaks the illusion being created by it
Movement Ensure the body moves in character with the mask at each moment. Techniques such as body tension, centre of gravity, rhythm, status can help interpret your mask's individual action style	Sound Any sound emanating from behind the mask, even a little sniff, breaks the illusion being created by the mask

(Continued)

Table 3.1 Continued

Technique	Obstacle
Audience interaction Make sure the mask constantly 'checks' the audience for response and 'shares' with the audience its discoveries. The technique is called 'clocking', using direct eye/face contact to ensure the audience is still engaged, like showing off, checking for a response	Mime Always use real props – real newspaper, real cups with real water. Miming a prop in mask risks being unbelievable
Audience placement Make sure the spectators are sitting 'end on' facing the stage. No one should watch from the side or the illusion is broken	Use screens or flats Never put the mask on, or take it off on stage in view of the audience. Use a flat, screen or turn away
Break the fourth wall and engage with the audience as much as possible	Consider your costume choices carefully or wear black

Excavation Four - building a character

Once the stance and typical gestures have been found, explore costume, props and objects. Start with large pieces of cloth such as shawls or scarves. In mask, find a way to incorporate the cloth – over the shoulders, round the waist as a belt, as a skirt, over the head, stuffed under clothing (Simon, Masking 44).

In mask, with cloth, play with a variety of real props from a props table – a rope to coil, knot or untangle; a trowel to dig and plant; a book in a foreign language; a stack of building blocks; a pack of cards; a chess set; toolbox; knitting; a puzzle. Present your props one by one to the audience. Take time to 'clock' the audience, showing the audience what it is, how much it is loved and what your relationship is to each one. Express your feelings about each prop.

Excavation Five - saying yes!

A prompter helps the mask to demonstrate various skills and actions by interviewing or auditioning the mask (for what job? Something incredibly challenging). Stay in mask no matter what. Listen to the audience to feel what is working and what is less effective. Say yes! to everything the prompter asks you to do or explain. Do it to your fullest ability, your very best effort, with sincerity, with passion, with energy.

Excavation Six – terrible twos conflicts

Here are some ideas for playing with the essence of drama - pairs conflict.

Dress an unwilling partner for an important date; teach a partner how to dance, wrestle, fence, sew, do tai chi; steal something from a partner (like props, hat or costume); two people on a park bench but only one has a real newspaper; movie goers at the cinema, one eating sweets noisily; in an exam room with papers, but one student has no pencil; lovers at a zoo; a tramp and commuter in a packed tube; artist and critic at an exhibition; newlyweds at a furniture showroom (Masks).

Compete with a partner to see who can do the chosen activity more, higher, faster, better.

In mask, develop a 'typical comic routine' or lazzo (plural lazzi, from l'azzione meaning 'action') for the mask. This is the default action - it could be as simple as a way of scratching the head and finding something to eat there; or as complicated as an entire comic routine. There is more to discover on creating a lazzo in the Commedia section to follow.

Setting the compass

Discuss these principles of mask:

Using real props and objects heightens the illusion of the mask.

The only measure of a successful mask is the reaction of the audience.

It's not just the way we are inside; it's also what we do and how we do it, which gives signals about our personalities and emotions.

Excavation Seven – interactions with other masks

The students have explored several different masks and now choose one to work with more extensively. They should start to build their mask in more detail now, providing details to the characterization. A character mapping chart like the one presented in Table 3.2 might help focus the different aspects.

Table 3.2 Character mapping organizer (Simon Masking 11)

Mask type	Shy looking, fearful
Name of character	Andy
Age	14
Facial characteristics	Eyebrows high and sloping down, tiny round mouth, eyes tiny and round
Key triggers	Looking for lost phone
Head	Tilted up, tilted to the side
Hands	Flappy, loose wrists, too big for the sleeves
Feet	Toes pointed inward, knock knees
Torso	Willowy, bendy, no backbone, wriggly
Shoulders	Hunched over
Hips	No hips, stiff, unbending

(Continued)

Table 3.2 Continued

Walk	Hobbling, falling over the feet, slow, clumsy
Stance	Hands at lower torso, wringing, legs crossed and twisted, shoulders hunched
Typical gesture	Hands flapping at wrist, arms hanging loosely
Lazzo	Looking for the purse in all the pockets of the jacket with no success
Central need	To feel safe and in control
Activities	Loves phoning and texting friends
Relationships with others	Online only, but intense
Emotions	Happy when chatting to friends, sad when alone
Thoughts	Can I make that person like me? Will I ever find someone to look after me?
Environments or surroundings	Bus stop, shop queue, urban lost in a crowd
More thoughts	I'm afraid of the big bad world and all the bad things that are bound to happen to me

Remember the rules of mask about facing front, not speaking or touching the mask, and engaging with the audience; the following exercises are spontaneous, unrehearsed, unplanned. Masks should enter the stage; 'clock' the audience response and react accordingly.

In groups of six to eight, enter with mask walk and present mask stance together in a line facing the audience. At any moment, prepare and start to sing as a choir, finish song, leave. It doesn't matter if the song is one word or more or never gets started.

In groups of six to eight, enter with mask walk and present mask stance together in a line facing the audience. At any moment, start a boy band choreography, finish and leave.

In groups of six to eight, enter with mask walk and ball and bat or equipment for a team sport. Sort out who plays what, where to stand and try to play. The rules of this sport are flexible and can change suddenly.

Resetting the compass

The mask reacts to the audience response. How does the mask respond to other masks? Is there a difference?

Excavation Eight - developing a scene

The following exercises (Simon, Masking 55-58) are led by the teacher, guiding and shaping the group. It is also unrehearsed and unplanned, as above.

Far away

In groups of eight to ten, enter in mask finding walk, stance and gesture. Masks find a place to sleep in a group on the floor. They awaken and gather firewood, build a fire and prepare breakfast. While eating breakfast (tasty/disgusting/too hot/uncooked/burnt) someone suddenly realizes a prize dog is missing. Everyone searches for the dog in vain. The group tries to think of a plan and eventually decides to hunt the dog by sled. Masks all jump on the sled to search for the dog. They find it, put it on the sled and bring it back to camp where they celebrate with song and dance. The masks feed the dogs and put them to bed, before stoking the fire to eat supper, recount the day's events in dance or song, and lie down to sleep.

Set the compass

Identify moments of believability in the performance.

Wilderness adventure

In groups of eight to ten, enter in mask finding walk, stance and gesture. Masks find a sailing or rowing boat and get into it, pushing it out onto a river. They drift and fish. A storm is brewing, and it starts to rain. The wind picks up, and the boat is plunged into rapids falling down a waterfall. Everyone is tossed out of the boat and has to climb back into it and get to shore. They tie up the boat at the shoreline on the edge of a forest and dry everything they can. They decide to enter the forest to look for food. They find a group of masks in the forest who share their food with them. The weather clears up, and they leave as friends, returning to their boats, waving goodbye as they go home.

Reset the compass

Identify moments of believability in the performance.

Excavation Nine – masked and unmasked

The interplay between actors who are masked and those who are not adds another dimension to the concept of identity, belonging or not belonging.

Whole-class masked performance to junior school level

Groups of five to six choose a picture book from the list of children's literature in the resources section such as Red (Hall), One (Otoshi), The Invisible Boy (Ludwig), Giraffes Can't Dance (Andreae). These are simple stories with stereotypical, masklike characters and non-masked individuals. The stories in these books demonstrate the power of being oneself, standing up to support difference and stop bullying as well as the power of bystanders to step up and support those being attacked (allies). Original masks can be made quite simply, and construction ideas are readily available online. Students should identify the action and any dialogue in the plot and thought-shower how they will bring the characters to life to send an important message to younger children.

Allow for discussion between actors and spectators after the performance.

Whole-class masked performance to middle school level

The Tin-Pot Foreign General and the Old Iron Woman (Briggs) provides a starting point for this ma performance. The work is set in the Falklands War, and Briggs draws a clear contrast between t stereotypes of power-mad, egocentric leaders, fighting pointlessly over possession of land – mine!' she screeched. 'MINE! MINE! MINE! I bagsied it AGES ago! I bagsied it FIRST! DID! DID! (Briggs) and the effects of war on the individual people caught between them. He does this th cartoon-like illustration that takes various features of both leaders and wildly exaggerates facial features (Dali-style moustache for the general; sharp, pointy nose for the British

Minister); elements of their jobs (power symbols such as general's cap and epaulettes for the General; huge hairdo, medieval armour and crazed eyes for the Prime Minister); elements of their gender (sword and spurs for the General; high-heeled boots and suspenders for the Prime Minister). However, when illustrating the ordinary soldiers and families caught in the battle and suffering loss of limb and life, the illustrations are suddenly pencil and charcoal drawings – hazy, without definition, ghost-like, nearly invisible, but human and individual. In groups of five to six, students read the story and discuss the illustrations. Thought-shower situations in the own environment that reflect two opposing sides of an important battle that can be stereotypically represented. This might be a battle between the Volleyball Club and the Dance Club to use the gym facilities, or it might be a battle between aspects of gender identity such as the 'masculine' colours and toys of childhood and the 'feminine' colours and toys of childhood.

Choose one scenario and clarify the intentions of communicating the topic to middle-school students. Develop exaggerated mask features for the two stereotypes on opposite sides that contain elements of job, facial expression, tools of the battle and so on. Thought-shower how to represent those caught up in the battle, those who suffer the effects of the battle, and those who are caught in the middle of the battle.

Create a scene with masked and non-masked performers to bring the message to middle-school students.

Whole-class reckoning

Social masks ease everyday life/social masks can cause harm.

A masked theatre performance, as an artist's construct (Craig 1957), has more power to move the audience's mind than mere actors without mask.

Resources, Full Mask

Andreae, Giles. *Giraffe's Can't Dance*. Orchard Books, 2014.

razell, Karen and Monica Bethe. *Dance in the Noh Theater Vols 1–3*. Vol. 1. Cornell University East Asia Program, 1982.

s, Raymond. *The Tin-Pot Foreign General and the Old Iron Woman*. London: Hamish Hamilton, 1984.

Edward Gordon. *Craig on Theatre*. Ed. Michael J. Walton. London: Methuen, 1983.

he Art of the Theatre. London: Heinemann, 1957.

harles. *The Expression of the Emotions in Man and Animals*. London: John Murray, 1872.

ul. *Unmasking the Face*. Los Altos, CA: ISHK/Malor Books, 2003.

Red. Greenwillow Books, 2015.

The Invisible Boy. New York: Alfred Knopf, 2013.

Trestle Basic Mask Resource Pack. St. Albans: Trestle, 2006.

t Everybody Is Saying. New York: Harper, 2008.

e. kokidsbooks, 2008.

Unmasked. Four Approaches to Basic Acting. New York: Palgrave Macmillan, 2009.

. New York: Palgrave Macmillan, 2009.

ese theatre painted face mask – erasing

atre in China, Xiqu, a form that includes singing, recitation, martial arts
ld. It has undergone many changes over time and there are strong
asic form is recognizably the same with singing, music on stage,

conventionalized movements, traditional stories and open-air performances to rowdy audiences. Among the regional forms, the best known is probably Peking Opera, also known as Beijing Opera or, Jingju. The term in Chinese simply means 'theatre of the capital'. The first Westerners to Beijing used the term 'opera' to describe the form because the actors do sing. But that is only part of the actor's performance technique. Other regional forms are Yueju from the Zhejiang area (see Chapter 5); Chuanju from Sichuan; Yueju (written with a different character) from Guangzhou and Hong Kong; Gezaixi in Fujian and Taiwan; or Bangzixi from Shanxi. In all these forms, not only must the actor learn all four skills – singing, recitation, martial arts and acting – there are also four key role categories, or types:

1. The male sheng
2. The female dan
3. The painted face jing
4. The clown chou

Within each role category are many subtypes: the male warrior, old male, middle aged male, young male; the blue-robe female, refined and demure; the brightly dressed, cheeky female maid type; the older female; the female warrior; and so on. The first two role categories, male and female (sheng and dan), use a type of powdered make-up that emphasizes their delicate features and represents their beauty and elegance. Neither of these roles is part of the tradition of the painted face, and they are simply known as 'handsome faces' or junlian.

The roles with painted face are either generals and military leaders (jing) or clowns (chou). When a child is chosen to attend the theatre school between the ages of eight and ten, the master allocates a particular role type to each student according to their stature, voice and face shape. Children with large round faces and big voices will be chosen for the painted-face roles while children who are good acrobats, cheeky, with a wide range of facial expressions will specialize in clown roles. A student will play only one role category all their life – in different plays, but always the same role type. In Jingju, the warrior or jing role is called the Great Painted Face (da hualian) and the clown or chou is called the Small Painted Face (xiao hualian).

Face score 'lianpu' - patterns in face painting and their meaning

In China, the written character used for 'face' (lian) has an important meaning beyond mere appearance. It also has connotations of reputation and social standing because it shows one's moral character. To lose face by behaving immorally or shamefully implies total rejection from the rest of society forever, to be outcast. In theatre, it is put together with the character pu, meaning 'score' in the sense of a musical score, graph or register. The term 'score' will be a useful one, since the face is painted with various different kinds of meaning all at once. In Chapter 6 of this book, we see how Robert Lepage uses the word 'score' for his theatre of interactive projections, where performance and production elements are layered to create moments of meaning.

The face score has been tailor-made for every individual jing or chou character in the Chinese repertoire. How each character's score is created has usually been developed over hundreds of years with minimal changes and revisions by actors, but it is always possible to know each character by their face score regardless of whether the play is being performed as Jingju, Yueju or Chuanju, just as the audience instantly recognizes Little Red Riding Hood through her red cloak and basket whether the performance is in France, Germany or Italy. The face score tells the audience everything they need to know about the character in terms of gender, status, age, personal life story of the character as well as traits of character. In this sense, it is a score of many different pieces of information about the character that the audience can easily and quickly 'read' from the moment the character appears on stage.

Painted face score: colour

The predominant colour of the painted face reveals something of the nature of the character behind it in a very general way. To every rule there is an exception, so these interpretations of colour must be taken in a very broad sense.

Red: it is the most important colour and carries the highest status. It represents a character that is loyal to the core, morally upright, righteous, brave and honest. Red also represents the yang quality of Yinyang – indicating male strength, virility, longevity (Riley 181–184).

Purple: it is closely related to the red face, dignified, cool-tempered, incorruptible, reliable.

Black: it represents characters that are more simple, rough and ready, loyal, bold, possibly not so attractive to look at, but faithful and reliable.

Blue: signifies arrogance, violence; can be cruel, cunning, cold, strong.

Green: signifies being brave and resolute, but wild, as if untamed, barbarian, like a forest outlaw. These characters are restless and easily irritated.

Yellow: represents a violent, calculating nature. Yellow faces hide their true nature under a rigid mien; they are generally of lower status, energetic, inexhaustible and often meet with a violent end.

White: whether powdered white as the face of high-ranking ministers, or oiled white face as military leaders, the whiteface is villainous and treacherous because the face is literally 'whitewashed' of all expression – the character is evil, hypocritical.

Gold and silver: these colours are reserved for gods and demons. They suggest immortality, and the ability to enlighten all those around by an inner aura.

Painted face score: structure

If colour is the first and most obvious symbol in the face score, then structure is the next. The way the face is divided and how different parts of the face are emphasized and shaped provides yet more clues as to the meaning of each painted face on stage.

1. Whole face

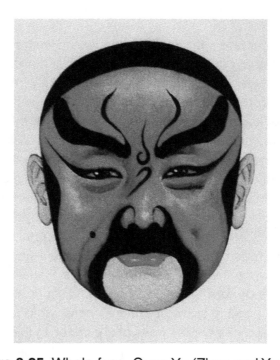

Figure 3.25 Whole face, Guan Yu (Zhao and Yan 43).

The entire face is painted in one single colour to represent a character of high status with a resolute personality, one who stands above any human inconsistencies, is a perfect person, nearly a god. The best representative of this face is Guanyu, of the Three Kingdoms period, still revered as lord of loyalty and righteousness (see Figure 3.25).

2. Three-tile face

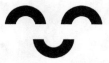

Figure 3.26 Three Chinese roof tiles.

Chinese roof tiles are laid in an overlapping pattern (see Figure 3.26). The three-tile face refers to the eyebrows and the bottom of the nose on the face. By dividing the face like this, there are three key areas remaining: the forehead and two cheeks. When a face is simply divided into these three areas, it is called a three-tile face. However, the three areas must be of the same colour. The three-tile face is most often used for characters that are good and kind such as Ma Su, who (somewhat overrating his own ability) volunteered to defend a strategic pass. Ma Su refused to listen to advice from the elders and made a rash move. The troops were forced to retreat with heavy losses. Although Ma Su had been a trusted friend and advisor, he was executed as an example, to show the importance of following orders. Ma Su's face has a narrow forehead and nose section to show the somewhat intolerant way of looking down on others. There is a red line running right down the vertical axis of the face as a foreshadowing of the execution to come (see Figure 3.27).

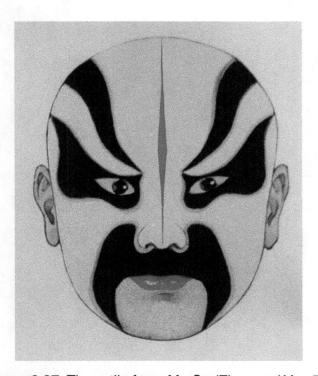

Figure 3.27 Three-tile face, Ma Su (Zhao and Yan 50).

3. Ornamental three-tile face

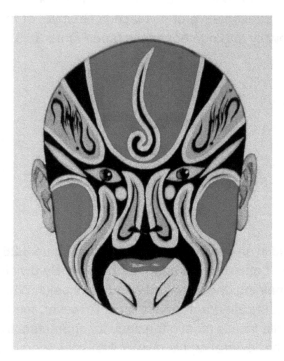

Figure 3.28 Ornamental three-tile face, Cao Hong (Zhao and Yan 47).

This face score follows the same colour pattern and structure as above, but the demarcation of brows and eyes is more ornamental. This is seen in the face of Cao Hong, a general who, although somewhat temperamental, was devoted to his leader. Cao Hong's temperament is shown in the wrinkled brow with its mark on the forehead to suggest a hot temper and irritability, and thinly demarcated eyebrows reminding us of the age and long experience of this character in battle (see Figure 3.28).

4. Shattered three-tile face

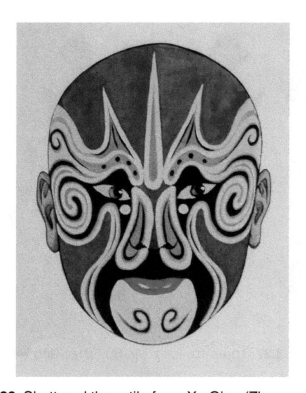

Figure 3.29 Shattered three-tile face, Xu Qing (Zhao and Yan 67).

The shattered three-tile face has even more decoration than the ornamental three-tile face, particularly over the nose. The more ornament and decoration on the three-tile face, the more the audience understands that this character is unsteady and probably not very calm in difficult situations. This is illustrated by Xu Qing, who helped to right the wrongs of corrupt officials (see Figure 3.29).

5. Shattered face

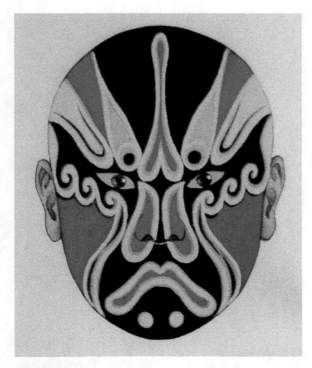

Figure 3.30 Shattered face, Di Lei (Zhao and Yan 76).

This face score is so multi-coloured and multi-patterned that the three-tile structure has disappeared. It indicates a hectic character that is powerful but with low status, someone who is very temperamental and changeable. The eyes are lost in the whirl of patterning, and exaggerated shapes as is seen in the facial score of General De Lei, who wielded sledgehammers in each hand (see Figure 3.30).

6. Ingot face

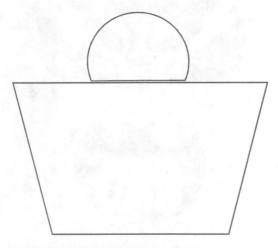

Figure 3.31 Chinese ingot shape.

Here, only part of the face is painted, and the painted part looks like an ingot of gold. A Chinese ingot has the shape of a small boat with a central dome rising up within the 'boat' (see Figure 3.31). The area above the eyebrow is not painted. These characters have malicious natures, but the unpainted, natural part of the face suggests that they have a conscience and scruples about their actions. Military leaders such as Meng Da (Figure 3.32) and Ma Han (Figure 3.33) are frequently allotted this face score.

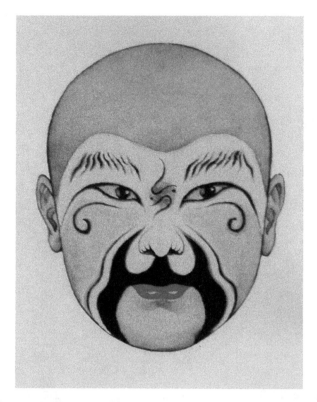

Figure 3.32 Ingot face, Meng Da (Zhao and Yan 44).

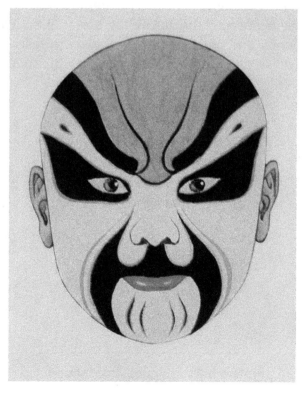

Figure 3.33 Ingot face, Ma Han (Zhao and Yan 65).

7. The character ten face, or cross-shaped face

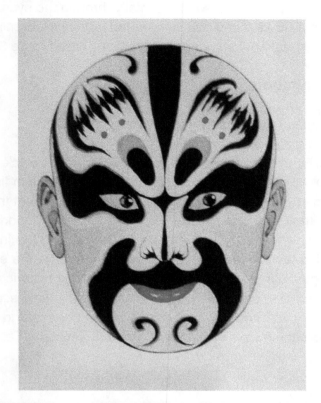

Figure 3.34 Character ten face, Zhang Fei (Zhao and Yan 43).

In this face score, the face is split vertically from the scalp to the top of the nose and on a horizontal axis that cuts through both eyes. The character ten is written like a cross: ＋. Typical of this kind of face is the loveable, cheery and good-hearted Zhang Fei (see Figure 3.34; Gissenwehrer).

8. Character six face

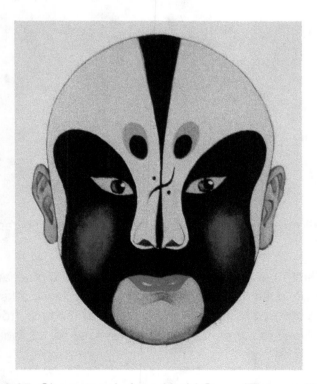

Figure 3.35 Character six face, Yuchi Gong (Zhao and Yan 53).

This face score is so called because the face is divided by the character for six: 六 vertically from the scalp to the bridge of the nose, horizontally through the eyes and then two diagonal legs around the mouth. This kind of face is interpreted by its most dominant colour such as the dutiful, brave, worthy official and old general Yuchi Gong (see Figure 3.35).

Painted face score: symbols

9. The symbolic face scores use objects integrated into the design.
    Butterfly:
    For example, Zhang Fei, pictured above in Figure 3.34, has a black character ten or cross face and the wings of a butterfly spread out as if about to take off in flight. The two points on the nose represent the eyes of the butterfly. The eyebrows represent the wings of a moth and run to a point where they turn into the sign for bat, symbolizing good fortune. Both butterfly and moth imply 'flying', which is part of Zhang Fei's name, and the insects are said to have extraordinary breathing techniques. Zhang Fei was able to blow the enemy away with fierce yelling and powerful gusts of breath. Legend dictates that the historical hero, Zhang Fei, had round eyes and brows like a leopard, also represented in this face score. The corners of the eyes are dragged down and nose drawn up so that the cheeks and cheekbones are high, small and rounded as if the face is smiling and cheerful, as Zhang Fei was said to be.
    Magpie:

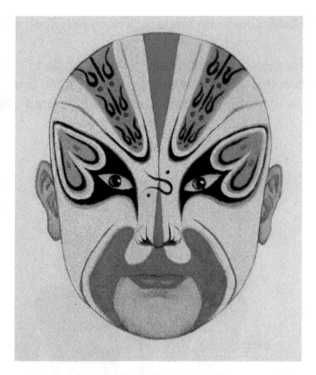

Figure 3.36 Magpie face, Tu Angu (Zhao and Yan 36).

The red markings reflect Tu Angu's bloodthirsty nature, and the cruel and merciless aspects of the character are shown in the tiny magpie eyes and black claw marks on the nose. Dark grey lines drawn below the eyebrows mark the musculature of the face, frowning to show evil, and the eyebrows themselves are surrounded in dark grey to show the fading age of the character (see Figure 3.36).

Magpie and Gourd:

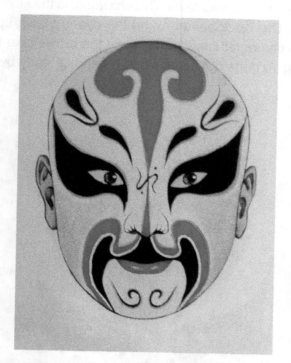

Figure 3.37 Magpie and gourd, Meng Liang (Zhao and Yan 63).

Meng Liang has a hot temper and loves to sound off. His face score combines a red character ten face with a magpie pattern, and a gourd. The gourd shape on the forehead and the red flames around the nostrils tell the story of Meng Liang's ability to light a fire with a calabash gourd. The gourd, or the winding vines of the gourd, are also echoed in the shape of the eyebrows. There are no round shapes at the nose, suggesting Meng is not a cheerful person, but rather somewhat serious and experienced (see Figure 3.37).

10. Steel fork face

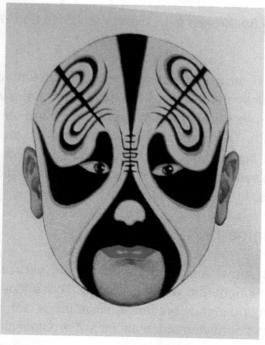

Figure 3.38 Steel fork face, Xiang Yu (Zhao and Yan 40).

This is a rare style of face reserved for only one key character, the Lord Xiang Yu, who can overcome any enemy and move mountains. This character is the key figure in the play 'Farewell My Concubine' (Chen). The black paint around the eye is drawn upside down, pulling lines downward, to show the character is suffering, while the brows take the form of the character for long life which Xiang Yu does not have, since he ends it early by committing suicide (see Figure 3.38).

11. Broken face

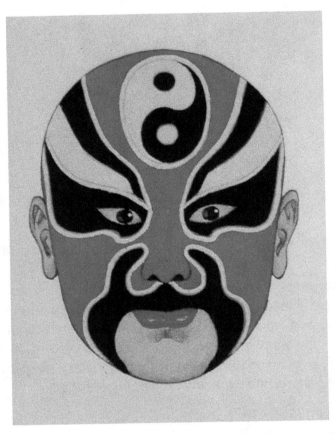

Figure 3.39 Broken face, Jiang Wei (Zhao and Yan 45).

These faces have regular structural patterns that are 'broken' by an image of something imposed on the face, usually the forehead like Jiang Wei. Jiang Wei was subservient to two nations and therefore carries the Yinyang symbol to show the ability to bring opposite forces together (see Figure 3.39). There are many broken faces on the stage; however, these are generally less important figures with less status and little to do on stage (little fighting or singing). The idea of one symbol branding a character is simplistic and should be avoided for more complex characters.

Painted face score: symmetry

All the faces described above are symmetrical on the vertical axis, indicating that their characters are basically upright and well-intentioned. Those faces with less decoration have higher status and a calm and steady presence, while those with more decoration have lower status. Those with crooked or asymmetrical faces are problem characters.

12. Asymmetrical face

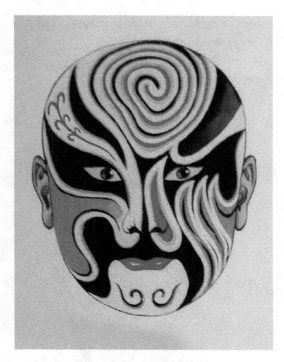

Figure 3.40 Asymmetric face, Zheng Zemin (Zhao and Yan 61).

Asymmetrical faces reflect that the character cannot be straightforward when mouth and eyes are formed in a twisted way. Many of these faces belong to murderers, robbers, executioners and evil military commanders such as Zheng Zemin (see Figure 3.40). Records of this historical figure suggest that Zheng has a twisted face because nothing in the world escaped his evil eye. Others suggest the twisted face represents an earlier battle wound. In both cases, the twisted face suggests that the positive nature of this character has been affected by something and turned into a negative, crooked one.

13. Asymmetrical face on broken structure

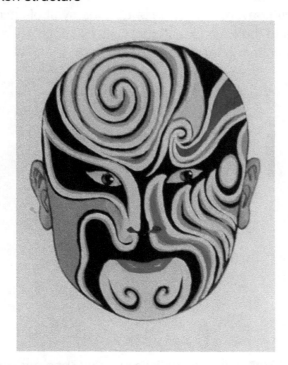

Figure 3.41 Asymmetric face, Qin Qi (Zhao and Yan 48).

Sometimes an asymmetrical face is adapted to show the character is not straightforward as here, where the mouth is twisted and the eyes at an angle. Asymmetry on a broken face structure is also used for murderers, executioners, robbers and unscrupulous military commanders such as Qin Qi (see Figure 3.41).

Painted face score: essence versus realism

14. Spirit face

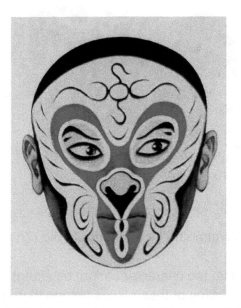

Figure 3.42 Monkey king spirit (Zhao and Yan 89).

Both gods (gold colour) and spirit faces have symbolic elements of the inner, essential nature of the spirit scored on the face. For example, Monkey King's face is not intended as a true likeness of a monkey as demon monkeys are. Monkey King's face contains an upside-down red peach for the stolen longevity peach, gold eyes after being burnt in the alchemy furnace for causing havoc in heaven, and a line of Buddha symbols across the forehead for bringing Buddhist scriptures to the East (see Figure 3.42). In contrast, a more realistic representation of a gibbon, a demon animal, is seen in Figure 3.43.

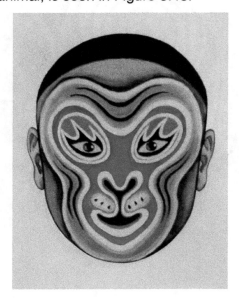

Figure 3.43 Gibbon, realistic animal (Zhao and Yan 92).

15. Demon face

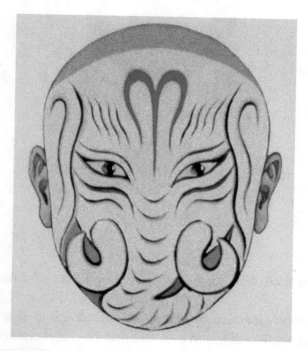

Figure 3.44 Demon face, white elephant (Zhao and Yan 95).

The demon faces more literally represent the animal being embodied such as White Elephant (see Figure 3.44) and Peacock (see Figure 3.45). These faces represent minor characters that appear briefly and do little on stage except add colour and spectacle.

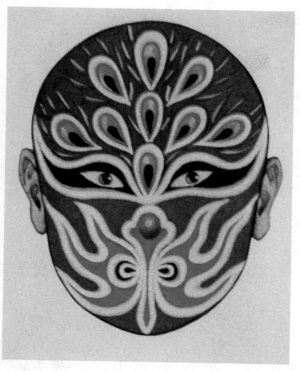

Figure 3.45 Demon face, peacock (Zhao and Yan 96).

Painted face score: age

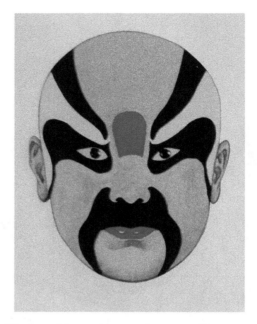

Figure 3.46 Aged face, Deng Jiugong (Zhao and Yan 87).

Older generals and military leaders show their advanced age in all structure and colour types by extending the white section between the eyes and ears and drawing the eye line downward to suggest the sagging skin of age as for Deng Jiugong (see Figure 3.46). The eyeline itself is sometimes drawn down to the lower ear lobes, and all vertical lines are softened and curved; there are no points or sharp angles to suggest youth. Sometimes, the eye shape is narrowed, and wrinkles are drawn around the eyes to suggest the poor eyesight of age and squinting to focus. Similarly, there may be rounded, shortened brows that wrinkle at the nose.

Painted face score: role type

16. Small painted face: the clown

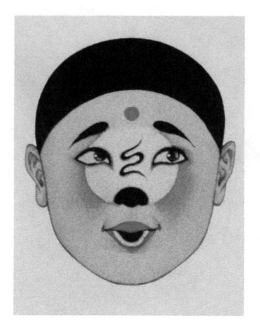

Figure 3.47 Clown face, cheery younger brother De Lu (Zhao and Yan 81).

The ingot face, above, should not be confused with the clown face, which also reveals some parts of facial skin. These faces are called 'dofu' or 'bean curd' faces, as if someone had thrown a block of jelly-like bean curd at the face. The bean-curd shape itself depends on each specific clown nature, such as cheerful De Lu (see Figure 3.47). The faces can represent old and young, and often evil or unscrupulous clown natures, including high-ranking corrupt officials, like Jia Gui (see Figure 3.48), and evil judges.

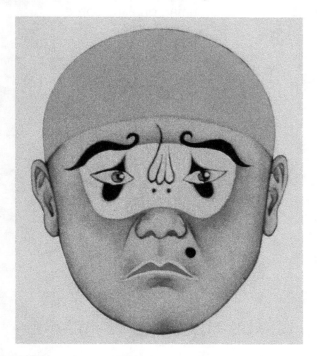

Figure 3.48 Clown face, corrupt official Jia Gui (Zhao and Yan 80).

17. Monks

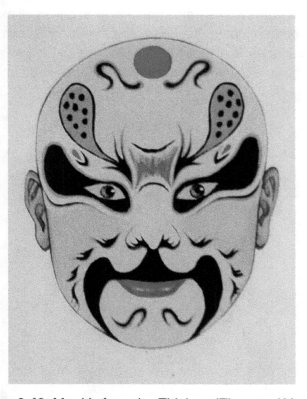

Figure 3.49 Monk's face, Lu Zhishen (Zhao and Yan 68).

These three-tiled, white-painted faces are generally marked as monks because of the eyebrows which are always in the shape of clubs, and eyes in the shape of kidneys because theatrical monk figures are nearly always warrior monks, such as Lu Zhishen (see Figure 3.49). Lu's face has the Buddhist pearl, a red mark in the centre of the forehead, and the red symbols between the eyebrows show that this monk still has many regular human characteristics. The black marks near the nose suggest a beard, for this monk is insincere – stealing away from the monastery to indulge in an all-too-human drinking spree.

18. Eunuchs

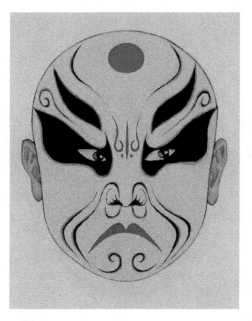

Figure 3.50 Eunuch face (with negative traits), Yi Li (Zhao and Yan 38).

Most eunuchs do not have painted faces because these are reserved for military roles. However, there are exceptions: some eunuchs do have painted faces and are recognizable as such by their willow-branch-shaped eyebrows, small round eyes and a small mouth (see Figure 3.50). A flame symbol must be present on the forehead, and the Buddhist symbol also used by monks is added to show that eunuchs do not take part in daily life. Liu Jin, for example, though a mean and cruel character, is given a red face to show just and unbiased behaviour (see Figure 3.51).

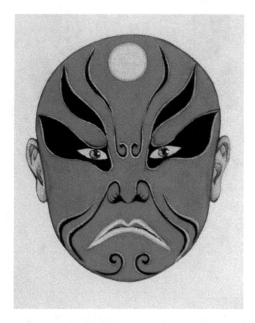

Figure 3.51 Eunuch face (with negative and positive traits), Liu Jin (Zhao and Yan 80).

Painted face score: character biography

Some faces change slightly in plays representing different episodes of their lives, or the character might be older/younger in different plays. Since many of the stories derive from historical records and fictional sagas, the structure, colour and creation of a face may vary, depending on the particular episode of the story being told.

Painted face score: details

Another way to read a face score of a character on stage is to look at the details of the eyebrows, eye shape, forehead, nose and mouth as separate systems of information.

Excavation One – paint your face

There are many videos online that show how Chinese theatre make-up is applied. Traditionally, it is always applied by the actors themselves; there are no make-up artists backstage. Learning to paint the face is a key aspect of training to act the painted-face roles.

1. On the website (Noll) choose a face created of three colours only – white, red and black.
2. Browse online for as much information as you can find on your chosen face, character and the play performed and document this.
3. Draw your chosen face on paper, noting how the lines dissect the face and where the lines meet ear lobes, nostrils, corners of the eye and so on.
4. Prepare your materials:
   Children's water-soluble face paint
   A calligraphy brush – with soft, shaped tip
   Mirror
   Headband or similar to keep hair off the face
   Sponge
   Water
   Tissues
5. The face is first sponged all over in white (unless the whole face is red).
6. Mark the lines in outline lightly in black. Hold the brush at 90° to the face. Pressure on the tip will create a thick line, while slighter pressure makes a very thin one. Draw the brush across the face starting with a thick line reducing to thin to get the sweeping-line effect around the eyes. Instructions on how to hold the brush are available online.
7. Complete the black shapes first.
8. Add any details in red and fine black.
9. Photograph your face and add some comments about how the shaping and colouring of the face made you feel.

Survey the terrain

Painting the face of the actor erases personal identity and replaces it with another.

Eyebrows: these can be natural, standard, old, dotted, slanted, one up one down, fang brows; wolf's tooth brows; duck-egg brows (bushy); wash-club brows (look like clubs); butterfly brows; silkworm cocoon, falling brow; arched brows, like a semi-circle; spoon brows; mono brow; long-life or swastika brows; gourd-shaped brows; heavenly bridge brows; praying mantis brows; and many more, such as flame, tiger-head, fine, willow branch, batwing, sword.

Eye shape: the shape of the eye may be standard, old, phoenix, birds-eye, ringed, evil-looking, drooping, kidney-shaped, gourd-shaped eyes, pointed, squinty.

Mouth shape: gold ingot, tiger, spirit of thunder, bowl of coal, water chestnut, drooping, crooked.

Nose: the nose might be rounded, pointed, black, grey, split, garlic nose tip, crooked nose, evil nose, laughing nose, flamed nostrils.

Forehead: a place for single symbols as in the broken face: Taiji symbol, northern star, trigram, flames, red Buddhist sign, tiger sign, long-life sign, sign for the eight trigrams, the calabash gourd, a rhomboid (indicating a bad end), moon shape (representing contact to the underworld), peach forehead (representing eternity), animal shape, human face, lucky sceptre, coins, halberd, Buddhist swastika, eyes, clouds, waves, the character for king, snail shape, gallstone shape, scar.

Whole-class reckoning

Colour, line, shape and symbols can distort, abstract, exaggerate and signify many aspects of status, character and biography to create a role. The actor's face can be scored with multiple textual layers of a character that can be read by the audience.

Resources, Chinese Face Painting

Farewell My Concubine. Dir. Kaige Chen. Perf. Fengyi Zhang Leslie Cheung. Beijing Film Studio. 1993. DVD.
Gissenwehrer, Michael. "Das Chinesische Musiktheater." '*Ich werde deinen Schatten essen*' *Das Theater des fernen Ostens*. Berlin: Fröhlich und Kaufmann, 1985.
Liang, David Ming Yüeh. "The Artistic Symbolism of the Painted Face in Chinese Opera: An Introduction." *The World of Music* 22.1 (1980): 72–88.
Noll, Paul. "Beijing Opera Masks." n.d. *Paul Noll*, April 2020.
Riley, Jo. *Chinese Theatre and The Actor in Performance*. Cambridge: Cambridge University Press, 1997.
Zhao, Menglin and Yan Jiqing. *Peking Opera Painted Faces*. Beijing: Morning Glory Publishers, 1994.

Commedia dell' arte

Commedia dell' arte was developed by small professional touring companies in the late 16th-century Italy, performing in towns, outdoor courtyards and marketplaces. The performances were loosely based on story outlines – scenarios – dealing with stereotypical everyday life issues such as young lovers being blocked by overprotective parents; older characters looking for magic potions to increase the contents of their purse, virility or long life and being duped; rivals fighting over a favoured love object; servants deceiving masters. The performances included improvisation, acrobatics, stunts, song and jokes. The half masks allowed actors to use dialogue, tone and dialect as well in representing specific characters such as the doctor, the lawyer, the captain, the lecherous old man, for example. However, higher-status characters were unmasked. The companies were generally all male, but over time females were included and took on the stock character of clever servant Columbine (unmasked) as well as the innamorata – female romantic lead.

Excavation One – stock character workshop

A stock figure is a stereotypical character that is easily recognized by everyone and has very little character development. In pairs, choose a stock figure from Commedia dell'arte and, using any or all of the resources below, create a workshop for your peers to teach them how to play your stock character. The workshop must include:

1. appropriate state of tension.
2. appropriate stance, posture, walk, gesture.
3. leading part(s) of the body.
4. characteristic animal trait.
5. lazzo or lazzi belonging to the stock character.
6. any vocal elements of the character.
7. information about the costume/mask/props typically used.

It might help to record findings on a table like the one in Table 3.3, working with a partner to add forms as they are discovered in a collaborative resource document.

Research organizer

Table 3.3 Research organizer of stock character

Tension state	Centre of gravity	Status	Stance
Posture	Leads with which body part	Walk	Character voice, dialect, tone, timbre, volume
Mask features	Costume features	Props	Animal trait
Speed, energy, dynamic	Lazzo or lazzi – comic routine	Acrobatics	Slapstick routine
Interaction with audience	Interaction with other masks		

A workshop planner like Table 3.4 might help to organize time and content.

Table 3.4 Commedia dell'arte workshop planner

Structure	What?	For how long?	Teaching aids
Introduction and focus of the workshop			
Activity 1			
Activity 2			
Reflection and wrap-up			
Sources used			

Excavation Two – identify and transfer stereotypes

As a whole class, thought-shower ideas for a set of six stock characters based on your own environment or community that all can agree upon, for example, drama teacher, teacher's pet, the nerd and so on. In groups of four, choose one of these stock characters to develop.
Following the analysis of stock characters in Commedia dell'arte, each group must plot:

1. appropriate state of tension.
2. appropriate stance, posture, walk, gesture.
3. leading part(s) of the body.
4. characteristics/animal trait.
5. lazzo or lazzi belonging to the stock character.
6. any vocal requirements of the character.
7. information on the costume/mask/props typically used.

Using the six universal emotions described by Paul Ekman, and adapting the mask in this chapter, each group creates a half mask for their stock character, and presents figure either through a video, like those used in the research section, or in live perform

Excavation Three – creating scenes

Remix the groups so that each group has four different stock characters. Quickly thought-hower a suitable scenario for the stock characters in the group and without any planning, play scene for another group. The scene must include at least one lazzo, one acrobatic skill, a fall, a joke and one musical interlude.
carefully, while performing, for audience response and repeat anything that prompts groan or gasp. Exit extravagantly.
eedback from the other group and repeat, making changes accordingly.

ckoning

ives and negatives of stereotype characterization in theatre performance and,
v life.

media dell'arte

haracters." May 2009. *YouTube.* April 2020. <https://youtu.be/7m6DjAHCWcY>.
2020. *BBC Bitesize Guides.* March 2020. <https://www.bbc.co.uk/bitesize/
.
e styles." 2014. *Theatre Links.com.* March 2020. <https://theatrelinks.com/-
he Routledge Companion to Commedia dell'arte. Routledge, 2014.
09. *YouTube.* March 2020. <https://youtu.be/ZUnaNTfTzuM>.
bazia cibo." April 2012. *YouTube.* March 2020. <https://youtu.be/

Excavation Two – identify and transfer stereotypes

As a whole class, thought-shower ideas for a set of six stock characters based on your own environment or community that all can agree upon, for example, drama teacher, teacher's pet, the nerd and so on. In groups of four, choose one of these stock characters to develop.

Following the analysis of stock characters in Commedia dell'arte, each group must plot:

1. appropriate state of tension.
2. appropriate stance, posture, walk, gesture.
3. leading part(s) of the body.
4. characteristics/animal trait.
5. lazzo or lazzi belonging to the stock character.
6. any vocal requirements of the character.
7. information on the costume/mask/props typically used.

Using the six universal emotions described by Paul Ekman, and adapting the mask templates in this chapter, each group creates a half mask for their stock character, and presents their figure either through a video, like those used in the research section, or in live performance.

Excavation Three – creating scenes

Remix the groups so that each group has four different stock characters. Quickly thought-shower a suitable scenario for the stock characters in the group and without any planning, play the scene for another group. The scene must include at least one lazzo, one acrobatic skill, a prat fall, a joke and one musical interlude.

Listen carefully, while performing, for audience response and repeat anything that prompts a laugh, groan or gasp. Exit extravagantly.

Absorb feedback from the other group and repeat, making changes accordingly.

Whole-class reckoning

Consider the positives and negatives of stereotype characterization in theatre performance and, by extension, in daily life.

Resources, Commedia dell'arte

Anderson, Samuel. "Stock Characters." May 2009. *YouTube.* April 2020. <https://youtu.be/7m6DjAHCWcY>.
BBC. "Commedia dell' arte." 2020. *BBC Bitesize Guides.* March 2020. <https://www.bbc.co.uk/bitesize/guides/zpfk6sg/revision/5>.
Cash, Justin. "Commedia dell'arte styles." 2014. *Theatre Links.com.* March 2020. <https://theatrelinks.com/-commedia-dellarte/>.
Chaffee, Judith and Oliver Crick. *The Routledge Companion to Commedia dell'arte.* Routledge, 2014.
"Commedia dell'arte Characters." 2009. *YouTube.* March 2020. <https://youtu.be/ZUnaNTfTzuM>.
Costola, Sergio. "AS2P Lazzi acrobazia cibo." April 2012. *YouTube.* March 2020. <https://youtu.be/VplfWbFosD0>.

Excavation One – stock character workshop

A stock figure is a stereotypical character that is easily recognized by everyone and has very little character development. In pairs, choose a stock figure from Commedia dell'arte and, using any or all of the resources below, create a workshop for your peers to teach them how to play your stock character. The workshop must include:

1. appropriate state of tension.
2. appropriate stance, posture, walk, gesture.
3. leading part(s) of the body.
4. characteristics/animal trait.
5. lazzo or lazzi belonging to the stock character.
6. any vocal requirements of the character.
7. information on the costume/mask/props typically used.

It may help to record findings on a table like the one in Table 3.3, working with a partner to add other terms as they are discovered in a collaborative resource document.

Table 3.3 Research organizer

Name of stock character			
Tension state	Centre of gravity	Status	Stance
Gesture	Leads with which body part	Walk	Character voice, dialect, tone, timbre, volume
Mask features	Costume features	Props	Animal trait
Speed, energy, dynamic	Lazzo or lazzi – comic routine	Acrobatics	Slapstick routine
Interaction with audience	Interaction with other masks		

A workshop planner like Table 3.4 might help to organize time and content.

Table 3.4 Commedia dell'arte workshop planner

Structure	What?	For how long?	Teaching aids
Introduction and focus of the workshop			
Activity 1			
Activity 2			
Reflection and wrap-up			
Sources used			

Crick, Oliver and John Rudlin. *Commedia dell'arte: A Handbook for Troupes*. Routledge, 2002.

The Drama Teacher.com. "Commedia dell'arte Conventions." n.d. *The Drama Teacher.* March 2020. <https://thedramateacher.com/commedia-dellarte-conventions/>.

Duchartre, Pierre Louis. *The Italian Comedy*. Courier Corporation, 2012.

Gordon, Mel. *Lazzi*. Performing Arts Journal Publications, 1983.

"Modern Day Arlecchino Examples in the Media." September 2013. *YouTube.* March 2020. <https://youtu.be/JkRPF90HiMg>.

"My Little Pony and Commedia dell'arte. An Analysis of Comedy." December 2012. *YouTube.* April 2020. <https://youtu.be/JuGTb3Lky34>.

National Theatre. "Commedia dell'arte Language." October 2011. *YouTube.* March 2020. <https://youtu.be/9gTs9xWJcgg>.

—. "Commedia dell'arte Shape." October 2011. *YouTube.* March 2020. <https://youtu.be/JJEwuurzDe4>.

—. "The World of Commedia dell'arte." October 2011. *YouTube.* March 2020. <https://youtu.be/h_0TAXWt8hY>.

Price, Lindsay. "Create A Commedia dell'arte Character." June 2015. *Theatrefolk the Drama Teacher Resource Company.* March 2020. <https://www.theatrefolk.com/blog/create-a-commedia-dellarte-character/>.

Rodriguez, Emily. "Commedia dell'arte Italian Theatre." 2019. *Encyclopaedia Britannica.* March 2020. <https://www.britannica.com/art/commedia-dellarte>.

Rudlin, John. *Commedia dell'arte: An Actor's Handbook*. Taylor and Francis, 2002.

Scala, Flaminio. *Scenarios of the Commedia dell'arte*. Limelight Editions, 1989.

Wilson, Matthew R. "In Plain Sight Ted Talk." November 2015. *YouTube.* March 2020. <https://youtu.be/PZFcl3MfgE0>.

CHAPTER 4

With gender – theatre history

The scramble for second-hand or vintage dresses and suits, two sizes too large and musty smelling; hand-drawn posters; giggles and sniggers backstage; and excitement for make-up of any kind. These are my memories of the annual school Shakespeare production, since drama was not a subject in the curriculum at all. And yet, drama has been part of most school curricula in Europe since at least 1540 when the Jesuits instituted regular performances by boys at their schools in order to learn to speak Latin and move with grace. The plays had a strong moral content. They were often stories that paralleled the real world, and the Jesuits believed that by 'playing' such model scenarios, children would learn about real life, social interactions, morals, politics and, of course, the values of religion. The same impulse drove amateur theatre at the schools and universities of Shakespeare's day. 'The clock struck nine when I did send the nurse'. Juliet's line rang hollow in my mind, and the teacher shouted. 'No, no!' I was simply not cut out for acting – for playing the nuances of this young girl waiting for news of her young, forbidden lover. I didn't have a clue where to begin. They say you have to be 60 to play Juliet well. Certainly, with no experience, no form to pattern my gestures and movements, no familiarity with the words of the text, though 14, I failed.

Drama and education are inextricably linked. Brecht created his Lehrstücke or 'learning plays' as educational experiences where pupils acted in pieces that challenged their knowledge of social politics. He wrote these model dramas as a space where events can be invented and tried out, tried on, discarded or adopted. A similar sense of modelling existed in the Jesuit school theatre performances. There were strict rules or 'conventions' about, for example, hand gestures. Franziskus Lang, a Jesuit priest, wrote down the rules of movement and gesture – a dictionary if you like – in 1727, and performances across Europe followed his pattern. It was like a universal language of gesture and movement. How to 'do' sadness' for example, or how to show 'rage'.

A convention is a useful tool in the theatre; like any rule it can be obeyed or broken. As this chapter will show, the conventions of what it is to be one gender, or another, were both consistently fixed and broken by European actors. Some of these devices were the result of laws prohibiting female actors from performing on stage, but it's clear that playwrights and actors also used the

DOI: 10.4324/9781003080800-5

concept of 'alternative or parallel world' idea of theatre to allow exploration of and playing with the outward appearance of gender, the movements and speech ascribed to gender, and the comedy and tragedy that can come about when the conventional rules of gender are broken.

Elizabethan theatre

Very broadly speaking, there were at least two different kinds of performance in Elizabethan times. The first kind was hosted by wealthy households where traveling entertainers performed. Wealthy patrons from these families financed the companies and thereby protected them from the usual penalties for traveling players and vagabonds who performed at market fairs. The wealthy patrons fought to have their theatre company perform at court as well. The companies were all male because females were generally not permitted to perform in public. The places of performance were any large space in a country house, court or palace. A second kind of performance was held in London and large cities, like Oxford, for example, at inn yards. The performing area was surrounded by balconies with rooms leading off them, making viewing galleries for spectators. James Burbage built and owned one of the first purpose-built theatres called the Theatre in 1576. Similar to later theatres such as The Rose, The Curtain, The Swan and The Globe, these performances were held in the open air all year round and designed like an inn with galleries and a yard. The stage is open on at least three sides of a raised platform, sheltered by a roof, the 'heavens'. The theatres were located outside the city limits in the entertainment quarters next to bear and bull baiting, prostitution and gambling dens. The stage had no backdrop or curtains to separate actors from the audience. Traps were used to make surprise entrances; otherwise, there was one entrance and one exit door in the back wall which was drawn from the Renaissance concept of the Roman stage. Food and drink were served throughout the performance, but there were no toilets. The audience sat on benches in the galleries or, for a price, onstage to be admired. The cheapest tickets were for the groundlings who stood in the pit or yard (a remnant of the bear/bull pit). The word 'groundling' derives not from standing on the ground of the yard but compares spectators to a kind of fish with a gaping mouth called a groundling. The Elizabethan performances nearly always ended in a joyful 'jig' with all the actors on stage and merry musicians creating a lively, cheerful atmosphere. This served as a 'bridge' into the everyday world, and performances at the newly built Globe in London (1997) continue this tradition.

Stereotype and conventions of character

A Shakespearian actor probably played several roles in different plays within a narrow timeframe. It has been suggested that there were so many lines to memorize, it would have been impossible to rehearse extensively and the actor may have resorted to 'theatrical shorthand' or conventions (Hyland 76). 'There would be comparatively little "theatrical business", and gesture would be formalized. Conventional movement and heightened delivery would be necessary to carry off dramatic illusion' (Bradbrook 109). Character types may well have had a set of rules or conventions that rarely changed: 'To work a comedy well, grave old men should instruct, young men should show imperfections of youth, strumpets should be lascivious, boys unhappy and clowns should speak disorderly,' says a contemporary of Shakespeare, George Whetstone (Bradbrook 53). Thus, the parts may have been similar to conventional role types like those used in the Commedia dell'arte. The performance occurred in daylight, in a rowdy arena, with wandering audience focus.

It is likely that standard, or conventional gestures were used to help communicate the role quickly and effectively (Bradbrook 21).

The queen's two bodies

By 1561, a common division of the given, human, mortal body (the body natural) and the public part being played (the body politic) is seen very clearly in the person of Queen Elizabeth I. She used this distinction in her famous speech at Tilbury. Though she has, 'the body of a weak, feeble woman' she also has 'the heart and stomach of a king'. For Elizabeth, the body natural was female, and the body politic was male, and this was a concept the Elizabethans could understand – is and is not – both at the same time. In the theatre at the time, females were not permitted to perform in public. The idea of two bodies might reflect the ability of Shakespeare's audience to suspend disbelief when watching young adolescent boys perform female roles (because the boys still had a naturally high voice). For the sake of theatrical convenience (changing costume), theatrical believability (the boy playing the female role plays a male character) for the sake of playing with gender (in comedy), or power relations (history and tragedy), Shakespeare created many female roles for boy actors that force them to disguise themselves as male for some parts of the play. Several kinds of 'being' are presented by a character in disguise: a boy actor playing a female role who disguises as a male. Taking the example of Queen Elizabeth above, where the two roles are understood to be contained in one body – an outer appearance and an inner nature – the disguised and undisguised roles in the theatre are superficial, external and conventionalized so that the audience can 'read' them without worrying about believability. In Apology for Actors, 1579, Thomas Heywood suggests that audiences are always aware they are not watching women, 'To see our youths attired in the habit of women, who knows what their intents be? Who cannot distinguish them by their names, assuredly, knowing they are but to represent such a Lady, at such time appointed' (Heywood 28). It would seem that these role conventions were predominantly dependent on the conventions of outward appearance (costume) and gesture.

What the audience knows

In performing a Shakespeare play, there is no backdrop or set, but, instead, actors describe their surroundings. 'Let us . . . On your imaginary forces work', says the chorus in the prologue to King Henry V, 'Think when we talk of horses, that you see them'. Not only the setting but also gender is created by simply saying it is so. Disguise is extremely popular in Shakespeare's plays. Sometimes a false beard, cloak or hat was enough to effect a disguise – in the disguise of boys in female roles, simply 'a skirt and petticoat' (Bradbrook 17). In the same way, Shakespeare's twin characters simply have to wear the same thing to be recognized as twins regardless of each actor's particular appearance. The audience perceives that the character is really a boy, playing a girl, playing a boy. This conflicts with the perception that the other characters on stage have of the role (the comedy derives from our pleasure in their ignorance) but there lies the drama! The key word here is 'playing'. The audience and the actors 'play' with roles and delight in the momentary suspension of disbelief. Later, Ben Jonson introduced a conscious appeal to artificiality by having the boys and actors enter the stage to discuss the play and their parts (Bradbrook 44).

Table 4.1 Four leading boy actors

Alexander Cooke, died 1614	Robert Goffe, died 1624	Salathiel Pavy, 1590–1603	Nathan Field, 1587–1620
Apprenticed to Shakespeare's company in 1597 and known for his performances of Lady Macbeth. Married with two children	Known for the roles Juliet and Cleopatra; married, one child	Trained at St Paul's before joining Children of the Chapel Royal. Ben Jonson wrote that though he was only 13 when he died, he was the 'stage's jewel' for three years	Famous for his Ophelia. By 1613 at age 26, he led his own company, Lady Elizabeth's men and was rumoured to have a child with the Countess Argyll.

Boy actors

There were two noted companies of boy performers: the St Paul's Company, who were St Paul's school choristers, and the Children of the Chapel Royal, also choristers, at the disbanded monastery of Blackfriars. These choir companies had been performing morality plays sporadically as early as the 14th century. The boys were trained in rhetorical-speaking and Latin. They performed in locations at court and in their own schools (a purpose-built theatre was built at St Paul's school in 1575) and ultimately joined forces and were very successful till about 1608 when they fell out of favour. Another kind of boy actor was an individual apprenticed to an adult company, and these were the boy actors for whom Shakespeare was writing. Boys between 10 and 13 years of age took on female roles while still pre-pubescent and their voices were still unbroken (Bottom, in A Midsummer Night's Dream, reminds us they should not have a beard yet). Shakespeare's company, The Chamberlain's Men, had two boy actors, one tall and one short, who played such pairs as Rosalind and Celia or Helena and Hermia (Hyland 2). Evidence suggests, however, that some boy actors continued to play female roles up to the age of 28 (Hyland 3). Table 4.1 shows some autobiographical details of four of the leading boy actors of the time.

Female actors

Female actors were permitted on continental stages, provided they were married. For English spectators, however, these female actors were like 'whores and common courtesans' who use 'immodest speech or unchaste action that may provoke laughter' (Orgel 3). In England, women did appear in public as dancers in court masques throughout the Elizabethan and Jacobean periods, but they were not professional actors, which was an important difference (Orgel 3). Officially, the ruling preventing women professionals on stage did not change until the restoration of the monarchy in 1660, when Charles II returned to England, having been exiled in France for ten years.

Excavation One – 'doublet and hose', 'skirt and petticoat' and 'young gentle'

As You Like It by William Shakespeare was first performed at the opening of The Globe Theatre in 1599 which bore the motto: *Totus Mundus Agit Histrionum* meaning 'All the World's a Playhouse'. In the two worlds of the court – where authority, law and religion dominate, and the forest – where nature, freedom and independence lurk, a series of love couples fall in and out of love. Rosalind is the lead – an unusual position for a female role – and she is banished from the court. For her own safety, she dresses in 'doublet and hose', while her companion Celia, daughter of another duke, dresses as her maid. Meanwhile, Orlando, also banished, has seen Rosalind at court and now wanders the forest writing badly rhymed poems about her and pinning them to trees. The disguised Rosalind catches up with up him and offers to pretend to be Rosalind so she can teach him how to capture the real Rosalind's heart. At the same time Celia falls in love with Orlando's brother; the shepherd Silvius loves Phoebe who falls in love with Rosalind in disguise as a boy; the clown Touchstone loves goat herd Audrey. Jacques, a misanthrope, loves and is loved by no one.

Midway through the play, Rosalind is invited to watch an argument between Silvius and Phoebe. She says: 'The sight of lovers feedeth those in love' 3.4.51. The drive of the play is watching couples fall in and out of love, as if by watching, the spectators might also experience love. The Globe motto, 'All the world's a playhouse,' reminds us that theatre is a smaller version (microcosm) of the real world (macrocosm). At the same time, there is double disguise for delight: Rosalind is played by a boy playing the role of Rosalind dressed as a boy called Ganymede, pretending to be the girl, Rosalind. The play is a perfect vehicle for playing with gender, playing with 'casting'.

In this play there are three generalized, conventionalized key role types:

1. The 'doublet and hose' role – physically strong, unbending, acts before thinking (see Table 4.2).

Table 4.2 Things we learn about the 'doublet and hose' role

Physical attributes and behaviour of the doublet and hose role		
'Because that I am more than common tall That I did suit me in all points like a man'? 2.1.110 'of excellent growth and presence'. 1.2 107 'Hercules speed' and a 'thunderbolt in the eye'. 1.2.188	'Proud and pitiless'. 3.5.40 The wrestling match in Act 1 The lion-killing in Act 5.1 Hunting celebration in Act 4.2 'Tears do not become a man'. 3.4.3	Of 'good conceit'. 5.1.52 (educated, refined, civilized) Respects hierarchy, law, authority (Duke Senior, reformed Oliver, Orlando)
Outward appearance		
'is his head worth a hat or his chin with a beard?' 3.2.192	'swashing and a martial outside'. 2.2.110	'sinewy'. 2.1.14
Props		
'A gallant curtle-axe upon my thigh'. 1.3.110	'A boar spear in my hand'. 1.3.110	'furnish'd like a hunter'. 3.2.230

2. The 'skirt and petticoat' role – passive, silent, distant, to be admired (see Table 4.3).

Table 4.3 Things we learn about the 'skirt and petticoat' role

Physical Attributes (somewhat unrealistic?) of the skirt and petticoat role		
'slender'. 3.1.96 More beautiful than a 'jewel'. 3.1.79	'Helen of Troy's cheek, Cleopatra's majesty'. 3.1.135	'Will not kill a fly'. 4.1.98 'Heaven filled her with all the graces'. 3.1.131

Outward appearance (very basic)		
'skirt and petticoat'. 2.4.8		
Behaviour (fades into the background – has no 'voice')		

'Her very silence and her patience
Speak to the people and they pity her'. 1.3.73
(Something that characterizes Rosalind is an
   endless ability to talk: 'Do you not know I
   am a woman?
When I think, I must speak'. 3.2.234)
	Faints when tired, 2.4.60,
	   and at the sight of blood,
	   2.4.70
	Changes colour when
	   emotional and at the sight
	   of blood, 3.2.169
		Like 'Atlanta's better side' (the
		   virgin not the huntress).
		   3.1.135
		Having 'Lucretia's modesty'.
		   4.3.168

3. The 'young gentle' role – young, unformed, changeable, uneducated, emotional (see Table 4.4).

Table 4.4 Things we learn about the 'young gentle' role

Physical attributes of the young gentle role		

'gentle, never school'd and
   yet learn'd'. 1.1.255
Gentleness is like being uneducated,
   naturally kind, in touch with
   emotions (what does education
   do to us?)
	'Your gentleness shall force
	More than your force move us to
	   gentleness'. 2.7.10
		'Let gentleness my strong
		   enforcement be
		In which hope I blush and hide
		   my sword'. 2.7.118

The feeling of lack of identity (feeling of nothingness, unformed, victimized by all)		

'If ever from your eyelids wip'd a tear,
And know what 'tis to pity and be
   pitied'. 2.7.116
	Empty, lacking identity: 'I shall do my
	   friends no wrong, for I have none
	   to lament me; the world no injury,
	   for in it I have nothing; only in the
	   world I fill up a place, which may
	   be better supplied when I have
	   made it empty'. 1.2. 170
	'Like a dropp'd acorn'. 3.2.220
	'as concave as a covered goblet or a
	   worm eaten nut'. 3.4.23
		The victim: 'Can I not say
		   'thankyou'? My better parts
		Are all thrown down; and that
		   which here stands up
		Is but a quintain, a mere
		   lifeless block'. 1.2.22
		'quintain' is a target for tilting at
		   in jousting

Changeable (emotions are not under control, appearance is out of control)		

'a moonish youth, grieve, be
   effeminate, changeable, longing
   and liking, proud, fantastical,
   apish, shallow, inconstant, full
   of tears, full of smiles; for every
   passion something and for no
   passion truly anything ... would
   now like ... now loathe...; then
   entertain..., then foreswear ...;
   now weep..., then spit . . .'.
   3.2.374
	'one inch of delay more is a South
	   Sea of discovery'. 3.2. 14
	   (impatient, impulsive)
		'a lean cheek . . . a blue
		   eye and sunken . . . an
		   unquestionable spirit . . . a
		   beard neglected . . . your
		   hose should be ungarter'd,
		   your bonnet unbanded,
		   your sleeve unbutton'd, your
		   shoe untied, and everything
		   about you demonstrating
		   a careless desolation'.
		   3.2. 346

The gap between a true/real self and a false/ideal self is called incongruity. Choose one of the role types above and create a Facebook-type profile for it on paper.

Flesh out as many details about your chosen role as possible: not just personal details like name, age, family, education, job, but also include ideas in pics, likes and comments that might be typical for this role as you would on a Facebook page.

Add the kinds of advertisement that might pop up on this character's page that a search engine may have generated from the kinds of website visited by the role as well as purchases made by them.

Now add a new page to show what's really going on in the 'true/real' idea of self, the authentic self of the chosen role. Draft some lines from a diary, or stream of consciousness.

Excavation Two – layers of identity

Create a short solo performance. Begin with an action that engages your role type (the false/ideal self) during the entire speech: dressing for a particular event; tidying, cleaning sports gear; repairing something that's broken; baking a cake; unpacking the shopping; building a shelf. In the first 30 seconds of your performance, you must establish the outward appearance and behaviours (conventions) of your chosen role.

How will you introduce the true/real self into the performance? Jot down some techniques that might help you: stepping in and out of role; projections; voiceover; inner soliloquy; interacting with other characters. You might find it helpful to map your ideas in four columns as shown in the organizer (Table 4.5). Where do these aspects collide? Where do they meet? Use highlighters and arrows to make connections and juxtapositions clear.

Table 4.5 Inner and outer roles organizer

	Thoughts	Appearance	Actions	Words
Outer role				
Inner role				

Excavation Three – war of the worlds

As You Like It sets up two clearly separate worlds, each with different rules and ways of being: the court and the forest. The court represents authority, politics, establishment, control, autocracy, injustice, cruelty, ruthlessness, spies, violence, urban, corruption, while the forest represents countryside, nature, freedom, self-discovery, democracy, equality, adventure, leisure, getting lost, topsy-turvy world, safe haven.

In groups of four to five, choose *one* of these worlds and transport the setting to an equivalent modern environment. The court might be turned into a parliament, a school, the military and so on. The forest could be a camping holiday, adventure holiday, a hike, travel to a foreign country, a rave, a theatre ensemble and so on.

Create three still images that clearly capture different moments of life in your chosen world. Make sure the essence of your environment is reflected in your shapes and use of space.

Without any rehearsal, two contrasting groups share at the same time, next to each other. Think, pair, share, then let the whole class reflect.

Each group selects one actor to play a role, as yet undefined. When Group 1 shares their piece this time, add dialogue and action. An actor from Group 2 must find a way to interact with the new scene as the 'foreigner', the character who is entering a new and different world or as the 'insider', a character who is familiar with the world and joins it easily. When Group 2 shares their sequence, the actor from Group 3 takes on the intruder role and so on.

Survey the terrain

Social pressure to conform to a particular way of being and doing things.

Excavation Four – shifting environments on stage

In the same groups, you must now create a physical set for your imagined world on stage. You should consider any items or props, live sound and use of space that Shakespeare had at his disposal, but you cannot use lights, projections or sound recordings. Once you have established your set, join with a group that is making a set design for a different world. As a group of eight, your task is to figure out how to move from one still image in one world to one still image in the second world as smoothly and as quickly as possible. Table 4.6 shows some possible techniques of transition on stage.

Table 4.6 Shifting the set ideas

Tell another story in a different spot while the scene changes	Actors move the set pieces as they exit/enter	Have the characters pronounce the location	Move the audience	Use notice boards or announcements like at a wrestling match
Black-clothed stagehands, like kurogo of Japanese Kabuki theatre (see Chapter 5), change the set while the actors continue to perform	Shift the action to a different part of the stage while the scene changes	Stagehands in costume relevant to the play move the set	Use screens (periaktoi), three-sided flats that can quickly be rotated to show a different scene	Use one table and two chairs in different ways for each scene as in Chinese traditional theatre
'in one' – a performer entertains the audience in front of the scene change	Kabuki drop – (see Chapter 5). Use handheld cloth to mask the change	Characters walk on the spot talking while the scene changes behind them	Throw audience attention to somewhere else in the theatre (entrance in the aisle?)	Create a choreography to move the set pieces

Setting the compass

All the world's a stage.

Excavation Five – the two Nats

'The Two Nats' is drawn from the book, *King of the Shadows*, by Susan Cooper. The book is based on the Shakespearian child actor from St Paul's School, Nathan Field (see Section Boy Actors). It tells the story of two actors called Nat. Nat[1] lives in 1599 and is about to play Puck in A Midsummer Night's Dream, with Shakespeare playing Oberon. Nat[2] lives in 1999 and has travelled to London from the United States to perform the same role in the same play at the newly constructed reproduction of The Globe Theatre. Magically, the two Nats switch time and place and learn about each other's worlds.

Dream of flying. Have students lie, eyes closed, in a darkened studio without touching. Run through some breathing exercises to induce a relaxed state. Read this passage very slowly with pauses, talking the students through the dream journey that will transport them from one world to the other, like Nat[2]:

You are at home. The hour is somewhere between night and morning. All is quiet around you; everyone is fast asleep. There are no other sounds in the room, just the quiet ticking sound as the digital numbers slip by on the alarm clock on the bedside table. As you lie, quiet, relaxed, feeling safe and warm in the dark, you slowly feel your body lifting from the bed. Your body rises from the bed through the ceiling, through the roof of the house and gently, slowly, feeling fine, feeling safe, you fly high, high up in the dark sky, past the clouds, up into the stratosphere, out into space. Space is dark and prickled all over with bright stars. Then you slow down, coasting and turning in space, as if you were swimming underwater; below you, you see the planet Earth, bright in the darkness, turning gently like a blue ball.

You hang there for a moment, and then you feel a hand take your own. You can see nobody, there is simply the feel of the hand. It holds you firmly, and pulls, and following the pull you dive down, towards the blue planet. It grows larger and brighter, and you can begin to make out the patterning of oceans and continents. Down you go, down, until you are heading into a white overlay of clouds.

> The hand draws you on . . . and into the next day. Your eyes are still closed, your body relaxed, but you know you are somewhere else. Roll to your side, still with eyes closed, gently come to a sitting position with eyes closed, kneel with eyes closed. Stand with eyes closed but imagine you have opened your eyes but do not open them. When I click my fingers, say out loud what you can see in your new world. What is happening around you? (adapted from Cooper 41).

Think, pair, share

How could you transport this dream sequence to the stage?

If the ensemble is ready for this, you could introduce Frantic Assembly's instructions on lifting and flying techniques (Graham and Hoggett 140f) and have them watch the demonstration at the National Theatre online (National Theatre). Make sure the students work in a safe, controlled environment.

Excavation Six – stranger in an old world

The world that Nat[2] lands in is completely different from the 1999 world:

> filled with people, bustling about, carrying huge bundles, selling fruit or pastries or pamphlets from trays slung around their necks, dodging to avoid men or horses. Carts clattered over the cobbles, creaking, rocking, splashing up muck sometimes from the stinking ditches . . . water ran through these ditches . . .squawking crows and ravens hopped and pecked and fought over garbage in the ditches . . . shop fronts where bloody meat hung on hooks, or vegetables and fruit were set out in gleaming rows, or a wonderful smell of fresh bread wafted out . . . people greeting each other . . . dogs snapping, beggars reaching out, a filthy child begging, hollow-eyed, stringy-haired beings with whimpering babies in their skinny arms. . . . (adapted from Cooper 52, 145)

In groups of four to five, create a small moving choreography of actions from this passage.
  In the same groups, now create a live soundscape for the scene.
  Now bring all the groups together on stage. First roll through all groups at the same time. Then, split the group members about the stage so the group members have to travel/shout/ keep eye contact with each other at a distance from each other, keeping up with the soundscape at the same time. Roll the groups all at once to make a cacophonous scene.
  Tag one random student to detach from their group and walk through the scene as Nat[2]. This student can tag another student to take over the role of Nat[2] and return to their actions as before and so on, a few times.

Resetting the compass

How could one add focus to the scene to avoid chaos? What tweaking does the scene need to be more effective?

Excavation Seven – intersecting worlds

While Nat[2] is in 1599 London, Nat[1] has been transported to 1999 to a London Intensive Care Unit, as he is suffering from the bubonic plague.

> Nat[1] lies half-conscious in bed, head tossing from side to side on the pillow. The wrists are tied to the bed by padded restraints, because Nat[1] has already tried to pull the intravenous line out – and that line, carrying fluids, nutrients and antibiotic drugs, is the only thing keeping Nat[1] from death . . . a Nurse, who has just been sponging Nat[1]'s thin fevered body . . . straightens the sheets, checks vitals etc. . . . Nat[1] can only see a pair of eyes in the Nurse's face covered by a mask, body in a sterile gown, hands in

gloves. Nat[1] hears a lullaby from somewhere . . . the scene is watched by the family, standing behind the glass, unable to enter the room. (adapted from Cooper 103–104)

Introduce the idea of crosscutting between scenes used in film and ask groups of three to four to quickly thought-shower and try out different ways to crosscut between the London street scene and the hospital. Share as whole class and try it out!

If the class would like to develop more scenes to intercut, here are some ideas:

A second whole-class scene in the streets of London 1599 as the population jostle to enter the yard of the Globe Theatre. What kinds of people are they? How much are they able to pay? They can buy ale and nuts and fruit from passing sellers; they chatter in anticipation of the play; comment on the spectators sitting in the gallery or on stage. A thief suddenly grabs a purse from someone's waist and tries to escape through the crowd. How do they react? What happens to the thief? The scene ends when the trumpet sounds showing that the play is about to begin.

Nat[1] wakes up in 1999 in the hospital not understanding any of the technology, surroundings or situation.

Nat[2] is standing backstage waiting to enter as Puck. What is happening backstage? Actors getting into costume, make-up and hair, eating, drinking, rehearsing lines, sleeping, chatting. Actors leave and come back. When the trumpet sounds, the play can start, and they exit backstage to enter the stage.

Nat[1] wakes up in the London hospital and is horrified at the meal served on the tray:

Breakfast first, said the Nurse and tugged a bed tray over my lap. Then you can have a shower – your clothes are outside the bathroom. Next to the door in the corner of the room was a small suitcase. 'Take your time, don't rush. Ring if you need anything.' There was a little buzzer on the bed next to me. The Nurse left the room. I looked at the breakfast tray. There was a carton of orange juice, with a small plastic cup inverted over it; a carton of strawberry yoghurt with a plastic spoon; a carton of milk; a carton of cornflakes; a paper dish, three little packets of sugar . . . a paper plate with two bread rolls in cellophane, two foil wrapped pats of butter and two tiny foil packs of marmalade, all held together on the plate by a roof of plastic wrap. I was looking at the result of four hundred years of progress. Still, I was hungry, so I ate everything that wasn't plastic, paper or foil. (adapted from Cooper 202)

Excavation Eight – safe worlds

In Susan Cooper's novel, Nat[2] has an aunt who seems to understand the comfort Nat[2] found in an alternate world – in this case, the world of the drama club. But the alternate world where one might feel at home could be any: the basketball team, a book, a film, a garden, a beach. . . . Take a moment to inquire of yourself: what would your ideal comfort – alternate world – look like, be like?

Excavation Nine – the end of the world

The end of the novel explores the theatre world as a microcosm (little model) of the macrocosm (the whole world). Remember the motto of the Globe Theatre: All the world's a playhouse! The character played by both Nats, Puck, steps out of character and appears as an actor for the final speech:

> If we shadows have offended,
> Think but this and all is mended,
> That you have but slumber'd here
> While these visions did appear.
> And this weak and idle theme,
> No more yielding but a dream,
> (5.1.412)

In the story, both Nats have been changed by the 'dream' experience. In groups of four to five, quickly devise an ending for the play of the two Nats. Will both Nats appear as actors on stage? Will there be a chorus, or narration, to explain what has happened? Will there be an abstract movement piece that recaps the transitions made by the two Nats?

Whole-class reckoning

Can there be two 'bodies' within one, like Queen Elizabeth? How can two apparently 'different' worlds come together – interweave, meld, clash? What might this say about the power of theatre?

Resources, Elizabethan theatre conventions

Bradbrook, M.C. *Themes and Conventions of Elizabethan Tragedy*. Cambridge: Cambridge University Press, 1980.

Cooper, Susan. *King of the Shadows*. London: Penguin Random House, 2010.

Graham, Scott and Stephen Hoggett. *The Frantic Assembly Book of Devising Theatre*. London: Routledge, 2009.

Heywood, Thomas. *Apology for Actors 1612*. London: Schoberl, 1841.

Hyland, Peter. "A Kind of Woman. The Elizabethan Boy-Actor and the Kabuki Onnagata." *Theatre Research International* 12 (1987): 1–8.

National Theatre. "Frantic Assembly Masterclass: Learning to Fly." 23 March 2015. *YouTube*. 4 March 2020. <https://youtu.be/Q4mXhW7TXQ8>.

Orgel, Stephen. *Impersonations: The Performance of Gender in Shakespeare's England*. Cambridge: Cambridge University Press, 1996.

The 17th century – men and women play women

First, a theatre timeline:

1576	First purpose-built theatre
1592–1594	Theatres close because of the spread of bubonic plague/the black death
1596	Puritans forced all theatres to move outside city limits

1603	Elizabeth I dies, King James I reigns
	Theatres close for another year of plague (30,000 deaths in one year)
1625	James I dies, King Charles I reigns
1642	Civil War between Puritan Parliamentarians (who wanted to remove the monarchy) and the Royalists
1647	Various bans and rules on performing theatre in public
1648	Playhouses and theatres destroyed; penalties introduced for giving public performances
1649	King Charles I executed, Oliver Cromwell leads the Parliamentarians
1649	Public performances banned entirely under Cromwell
1658	Cromwell dies, Puritans lose hold. Theatres resurge
1660	Restoration of the monarchy – King Charles II returns from exile in France
1688	King Charles II dies

What a tumultuous time for theatre! How closely theatre performances are linked to the politics, religion, even health of the society of the time! Even now, around the world, performances are censored, shaped or banned by religious and/or political strictures. And in 2020, theatres and cinemas closed because of the fear of spreading the SARS Covid-19 virus.

Although upper class, aristocratic ladies certainly took part in Elizabethan and Jacobean court masque, such as the singers Madame Coniak and Mistress Shepard (Orgel 5), it was considered improper for women to perform professionally on stage. The film 'Shakespeare in Love' treats this theme with much imagination and charm. As soon as the monarchy was restored when King Charles II returned from exile in France, theatres began to flourish once more; old theatres were revived, and new ones built. And one thing King Charles brought back from the French court was the idea that female professional actors were not only acceptable, but also desirable, to avoid any indecency suggested by boys playing women. The repertoire of Restoration drama largely consisted of aristocratic comedies of intrigue, comedies of manners, poking fun with satirical and quick-witted dialogue at the self-absorbed, artificial and fashion-driven aristocracy. Of course, Shakespeare and the other classics were also performed – sometimes with a changed, happier ending.

Gender fluidity in the turbulent 1600s

Not forgetting the two bodies of Queen Elizabeth I having the body of a woman but the heart of a king, throughout art, court life and the theatre, there is much evidence of playing with the outward appearance of gender. The strong female, the huntress amazon, was a 'role' frequently presented by women in positions of political power. For example in 1617 Paul van Somer painted a portrait of Queen Anne, wife of James I, wearing a riding costume which everyone knew by the French term 'amazon' (Orgel 87). Similarly, portraits of Elizabeth Carey and Elizabeth of Bohemia show them wearing armour and a 'doublet'. Rosalind may only have needed to change a skirt for hose! Charles I himself performed in a masque in 1640 in a role associated with 'Hermaphroditus, the youth who never attains (adult, patriarchal) autonomy but rather . . . at once, effeminate youth and wanton woman, the sexual attributes of each mapped on a single body' (King 63). But these roles were played at court by aristocrats, not professional actors; the audience was noble, not common. Similarly, King James complained about women wearing masculine broad-brimmed hats, pointed doublets and hair cut or shorn. On the public, professional stage, there is an account of a performance of Desdemona's death scene in Othello in 1610 where

her face alone implored the pity of the audience . . . are we not entitled to assume from this . . . that the men who played women could act anything demanded of them, without the need to formalize or symbolize their actions, to disguise their age or their sex? (Hyland 6)

Thomas Heywood felt it was unlawful to cross-dress in real life, while on the stage everyone knows it's just a role: 'Who cannot distinguish them by their names, assuredly knowing they are but to represent such a lady, at such a time appointed?' (Heywood 28).

Ned Kynaston (*c.*1640-1706), male actor of female roles

In anticipation of the restoration of the monarchy, several entrepreneurs moved to open theatre companies in London between May 1659 and March 1660. By 1660 there were still some male actors specializing in female roles performing on stage. One of these was Ned Kynaston who was said to have 'something of a formal Gravity in his mien, which was attributed to the stately Step' he had learned from performing female roles (Heywood 72). Others commented that his performance of women had 'disagreeable tones in speaking, something like whining, or what we term canting' (King 260). On one occasion, a contemporary reports that King Charles arrived at the theatre too early. The theatre manager decided to tell the truth and explain that the Queen (played by Kynaston) 'was not shav'd yet' (Haggerty 309). Samuel Pepys, the great diarist, wrote of Kynaston that he 'made the loveliest lady that ever I saw in my life, only her voice was not very good' (Hyland 311). A third source even claims that female actors performing the same part could not compare with him since he was 'very Young, and Made a Complete Female Stage Beauty, performing his Parts so well . . . that it has since been Disputable among the judicious, whether any woman that succeeded him so Sensibly touch'd the audience as he' (Hyland 313). John Downes, a contemporary, listed the parts Kynaston played each season (Downes 19) from 1660 to 1662. Included in this list is the title role of a play by Ben Jonson – Epicene or The Silent Woman, where Kynaston also played a male role. The main character in this comedy is in disguise as a woman until the very end of the play, when she is revealed to be a 'he'. Samuel Pepys notes that Kynaston appeared 'in fine clothes as a gallant, and in them was clearly the prettiest woman in the whole house – and . . . as a man; and then likewise did appear the handsomest man in the house' (Hyland 314). Later, Kynaston also played the role of Sir Dauphine, who exposes Epicene to be a man underneath by whisking off her wig. Having played a woman who was really a man in this play, Kynaston similarly starred in Jonson's play Volpone as a man who is 'really' a woman. He retired aged 42 in 1698. Other male actors of the time also continued to play female roles before switching to male roles, among them Edward Angel, who later became a popular low comedian (Downes 154), and James Nokes, John Honyman, Theosophilus Bird and Charles Hart (Downes 19).

Margaret Hughes (*c.*1645-1719), female actor of female roles

Mrs Margaret Hughes was possibly the first female actor on the English public stage in 1660 since some suggest it was she who was listed as performing Desdemona in Othello (Downes 78). Other sources suggest the actor was her rival, Anne Marshall. A Prologue and Epilogue was added to this performance by Thomas Jordan. He opens the prologue by saying he has seen the actor getting dressed backstage and can verify it is a genuine woman, not a man in a petticoat. He says he 'knows' her, suggesting he has had sexual relations with her, but requests the audience to respect that she is virtuous. He warns them not to wait for her backstage as this would be improper. Most of this sounds like a direct invitation to view the actor as sexually available after the show, however. After the performance, the epilogue asks 'how d'ye like her', another double entendre, and suggests the success or lack of success is in the spectator's 'hands' (Ritchie). The diarist, Samuel Pepys thought Margaret Hughes was a 'pretty woman' whom he may have kissed backstage (Highfill, Burnim and Langhans 24) with 'dark ringleted hair, a fine figure, and particularly good legs' (Spencer 218). The new playwrights such as Fletcher, Beaumont, Massinger and others started to explore a wider range of female roles than those 'silent women' and 'boy actors' found in Shakespeare, such as the 'noble harlot' and 'villainess'. In fact, nearly one-fourth of all plays now contained one or more cross-dressed parts (female actors in female roles impersonating male roles) and 14 plays featured female actors in male roles (Ritchie 35). Where a female actor was playing a male role whether cross-dressed or in travesty, the role was known as 'breeches role'; the aim of which was certainly to show off the female body and not to impersonate the male. A portrait of Margaret Hughes by Sir Peter Lely in 1670 shows her left breast completely exposed, highlighting features other than her good acting.

Anne Bracegirdle, 1663-1748

Anne, coached by actor and theatre manager Thomas Betterton, was a favourite with spectators, not least because of her appearance,

> She was of lovely height, with dark brown hair and eyebrows, black sparkling eyes and fresh blushy complexion, and whenever she exerted herself had an involuntary Flushing in her Breast, Neck and Face, having continually a cheerful aspect and a fine set of white teeth. (Nagler 128)

Her specialty was comedy, where she was said to excel particularly playing male roles where a long wig could cover her only defect, a slightly hunched shoulder. Typical of several records of female actors of the time, the report focuses almost exclusively on physical attributes, 'she was finely shaped and had very handsome legs and feet and her gait or walk was free, manlike and modest when in breeches' (Nagler 130).

Other female actors included Elizabeth Barry, Mrs Davenport, Mrs Davies, Mrs Saunderson (known for playing Ophelia), Mrs Long (known for playing Dulcino the Grateful Servant in male costume), Mrs Ann Gibbs, Mrs Holden, Mrs Norris, Mrs Jennings (Downes 20–27). Mrs Charlotte Clarke was the daughter of theatre manager, Colley Cibber, who fell into poverty and wrote a small memoir (Clarke). Similar autobiographies exist by Mrs Ann Oldfield, a 'celebrated actress' (Oldfield) and Margaret Woffington, who describes her appearance as Harry Wildair (Woffington). Some female actors were hired from the Continent: dancers and singers such as Madame Delphine earned 10,000 Guineas (Downes 46). Significant early female playwrights include Aphra Behn, Mary Pix and Catherine Trotter (O'Quinn, Straub and Anderson; Nussbaum).

Excavation One – I don't know how to do it!

Read the poem 'For Ezekiel Fenn at his first acting a man's part' (Glapthorne) shown in Table 4.7.

Ezekiel (c.1620) was known for performing demanding female roles (Banham 341). The poet suggests that Ezekiel's first performance in a male role was a disaster, however, so he begs the reader to give the actor more time to learn how to play 'as a man'.

Think, pair, share

What do you think Ezekiel did 'wrong'?

Table 4.7 Poem for Ezekiel Fen with modern version (Glapthorne)

For Ezekiel Fen at his first Acting a Man's Part by Henry Glapthorne (1639)	Modern version:
Suppose a Merchant when he launches forth An untried vessel, doubtful of its worth, Dare not adventure on that infant piece The glorious fetching of a golden fleece From the remotest Indies. 'Tis so with me, Whose innocence and timerous modesty Does blush at my own shadow, prone to fear Each wave a billow that arises here; The company's my merchant nor dare they Expose my weak frame on so rough a sea, 'Less you (their skilful pilots) please to steer By mild direction of your eye and ear Their new rigg'd bark. This is their hope and mine Promise my selfe; if you like north-stars shine, I like a daring, and adventrous man, Seeking new paths i'th' angry ocean, In threatning tempests, when the surges rise And give salt kisses to the neighb'ring skies, When blustring *Boreas* with impetuous breath Gives the spread sails a wound to let in death, Cracks the tall mast, forcing the ship (though loathe) On its carv'd prow to wear a crown of froth; Will face all perils boldly, to attain Harbour in safety; then set forth again.	If a merchant trader chose to launch a boat that's never been tested before, they wouldn't send it out on a huge journey to the Indies. I'm like that untested boat, because I am still innocent and shy and blush at my own shadow. I would be terrified of every wave that crashes over the edge. The theatre company is like the merchant trader and the ensemble leader doesn't dare to let me loose on the rough water of the stage unless you, dear audience, by using your eyes and ears, are willing to help steer me in the right direction. If you are willing, then I will be adventurous and try my best even when the sea is raging, and the wind is blasting in my face. I will sail into the harbour and then, with this experience, go back on stage and try again.

Excavation Two – playing woman, playing man

The film, Stage Beauty (Hatcher), is a fictional account of the rise of female actors onstage during the Restoration period and the fall of male actors of female roles. It is based on real-life historical figures Ned Kynaston and Margaret Hughes and is a good resource for looking at courtly stages and public theatres of the time as well. If you cannot watch the whole film to provide background about the conventional gestures of femininity used at the time watch these following scenes:

1. Kynaston teaches Mrs Hughes the five positions of female subjugation 039.09–040.00.
2. Kynaston attempts to play Othello 1:04:24–1:09.00.

In groups of three, complete the tables of outward appearance (Table 4.8), gestures of the actor (Table 4.9) and voice (Table 4.10) as you watch the two performances of Desdemona by Kynaston and Mrs Hughes.

1. Kynaston performs Desdemona in the 'traditional style' 0:00:00–0:04:00.
2. Mrs Hughes performs Desdemona in a more 'naturalistic' style of acting 1:27:00–1:40:00.

Table 4.8 Comparing the outward appearance of two actors

Outward appearance of the actor	'Kynaston'	'Margaret Hughes'
Costume		
Make-up		
Hair		
Props		

Table 4.9 Comparing the gestures used by both actors

Gesture of the actor	'Kynaston'	'Margaret Hughes'
Hand(s)		
Body shapes and movement		
Feet		

Table 4.10 Comparing the voice used by both actors

Voice	'Kynaston'	'Margaret Hughes'
Tone		
Timbre		
Breath		

Survey the terrain

What reflections and conclusions can you draw about 'playing' gender? In your groups, map your thoughts using any of the ideas shown in Table 4.11.

Table 4.11 Different ways to reflect on playing gender

Role: as director on Othello, if you were directing Kynaston as Desdemona, or if you were directing Margaret, what instructions would you give? Would they be different?	Five Times Why: start with a why question and chain four more questions to your answer.	Clustering – scribble all thoughts down before linking them with highlighters, arrows, overlaps and so on.	Create a spider web of responses as you observe the scene.
What if? Imagine you were in Kynaston or Margaret's shoes? How would you feel?	Mind map – create a mind map starting from one moment in the death scene.	Use de Bono's six thinking hats: Blue – The big picture; White – Facts and information;	Thought-shower a famous person in history and imagine how they would handle the performance.

(Continued)

Table 4.11 Continued

		Red – Feelings and emotions; Black – Critical judgement; Yellow – Positive ideas Green – New ideas.	
Identify SWOT (Strengths, Weaknesses, Opportunities, Threats).	Starbursting (write down the issue in the centre and then at each tip of the star, who, what, where, why, when, how, to reflect).	Reverse brainstorming (identify the causes of the problem).	Slip Writing (grab a pad of stickies and write at least five thoughts. Pin, share, add to other people's stickies.

Excavation Three – 'Blind' casting

Contemporary theatre practice allows for all actors to be considered for all roles regardless of ethnicity, skin colour, body shape, age or or gender. It is a policy much argued, however (see the discussion of the yellow-facing of Jonathan Pryce in Miss Saigon or casting black actors as George Washington and Thomas Jefferson in the musical Hamilton). 'Blind' gender casting in theatre, however, is seen as a way to explore the intricacies and complexities of a role, to cast the role in a new light. Fiona Shaw playing Richard II in 1996; Phyllida Lloyd's all-female cast performing Julius Caesar at the Donmar Warehouse in 2012; Mark Rylance's 'Original Practice' at the Globe Theatre in an all-male Twelfth Night in 2012; and Emma Rice's version of A Midsummer Night's Dream at the Globe in 2018 are just a few examples.

In the Elizabethan and Restoration theatres, the audience was aware of the gender of the actor and accepted certain conventions of gesture or appearance.

In pairs, take a few lines from the Desdemona and Othello dialogue below and explore adopting the appearance, movement and voice of another gender in performance. Explore several different combinations.

Act 5 Scene II. A bedchamber in the castle: Desdemona in bed asleep; a light burning.
Enter Othello

DESDEMONA: Who's there? Othello?
OTHELLO: Ay. Desdemona.
DESDEMONA: Will you come to bed, my lord?
OTHELLO: Have you pray'd to-night, Desdemona?
DESDEMONA: Ay, my lord.
OTHELLO: If you bethink yourself of any crime
Unreconciled as yet to heaven and grace,
Solicit for it straight.
DESDEMONA: Alas, my lord, what do you mean by that?

OTHELLO: Well, do it, and be brief; I will walk by:
            I would not kill thy unprepared spirit;
            No; heaven forfend! I would not kill thy soul.
DESDEMONA: Talk you of killing?
OTHELLO: Ay, I do.
DESDEMONA: Then heaven Have mercy on me!
OTHELLO: Amen, with all my heart!
DESDEMONA: If you say so, I hope you will not kill me.

. . .

OTHELLO: Think on thy sins.
DESDEMONA: They are loves I bear to you.
OTHELLO: Ay, and for that thou diest.
DESDEMONA: That death's unnatural that kills for loving.
            Alas, why gnaw you so your
            nether lip?
            Some bloody passion shakes your very frame:
            These are portents;
            but yet I hope, I hope,
            They do not point on me.
OTHELLO: Peace, and be still!
DESDEMONA: I will so. What's the matter?
OTHELLO: That handkerchief which I so loved and gave thee
            Thou gavest to Cassio.
DESDEMONA: No, by my life and soul!
            Send for the man, and ask him.
OTHELLO: Sweet soul, take heed, Take heed of perjury;
            thou art on thy deathbed.

. . .

DESDEMONA: Then Lord have mercy on me!
OTHELLO: I say, amen.

. . .

DESDEMONA: O, banish me, my lord, but kill me not!
OTHELLO: Down, strumpet!
DESDEMONA: Kill me to-morrow: let me live to-night!
OTHELLO: Nay, if you strive -
DESDEMONA: But half an hour!
OTHELLO: Being done, there is no pause.
DESDEMONA: But while I say one prayer!
OTHELLO: It is too late.

He stifles her

Whole-class reckoning

Is femininity performed differently by women and men? Is masculinity performed differently by women and men? What are the positives and negatives of cross-gender-casting?

Resources, men and women play women

Banham, Martin, ed. *The Cambridge Guide to World Theatre*. Cambridge: Cambridge University Press, 1990.

Clarke, Charlotte. *Narrative of the Life of Mrs. Charlotte Clarke*. Ed. Leonard Ashley. London: Gainsville scholar's facsimiles and reprints, 1969.

Downes, John. *Roscius Anglicanus*. Ed. Montague Summers. Robarts University of Toronto, 1928.

Haggerty, George E. "'The Queen was not shav'd yet': Edward Kynaston and the Regendering of the Restoration Stage." *The Eighteenth Century* 50.4 (2009): 309–326.

Heywood, Thomas. *Apology for Actors 1612*. London: Schoberl, 1841.

Highfill, Philip H., Kalman A. Burnim, and Edward A. Langhans. *A Biographical Dictionary of Actors, Actresses, Musicians, Dancers, Managers and Other Stage Personnel in London 1660–1800*. Vol. 8. Carbondale: Southern Illinois University Press, 1982.

Hyland, Peter. "'A kind of woman' the Elizabethan Boy-Actor and the Kabuki Onnagata." *Theatre Research International* 12 (1987): 1–8.

Glapthorne, Henry. *The Plays and Poems of Henry Glapthorne: The tragedy of Albertus Wallenstein*. The ladies priviledge. Poems. London: John Pearson, 1874. 196.

King, Thomas A. The Gendering of Men 1600–1750, Vol. 2, Queer Articulations. Madison: University of Wisconsin Press, 2008.

Nagler, A. *A Source book in Theatrical History*. New York: Dover, 1952.

Nussbaum, Felicity. *Rival Queens: Actresses, Performance and the Eighteenth-Century British Theater*. Philadelphia: University of Pennsylvania Press, 2010.

O'Quinn, Daniel, Kristina Straub, and Misty G. Anderson. *The Routledge Anthology of Restoration and Eighteenth-Century Performance*. London: Routledge, 2019.

Oldfield, Ann. *The Authentic Memoirs of the Life of that Celebrated Actress Mrs Ann Oldfield*. London: Printed, and sold by the booksellers and pamphlet sellers of London and Westminster, 1730.

Orgel, Stephen. *Impersonations: The Performance of Gender in Shakespeare's England*. Cambridge: Cambridge University Press, 1996.

Ritchie, Fiona. *Women and Shakespeare in the 18th Century*. Cambridge: Cambridge University Press, 2014.

Spencer, Charles. *Prince Rupert: The Last Cavalier*. London: Phoenix, 2007.

Stage Beauty. By Jeffrey Hatcher. Dir. Richard Eyre. Perf. Billy Crudup, Clare Danes and Rupert Everett. Lions Gate Films. 2004. DVD.

Woffington, Mary. *Memoirs of the Celebrated Mrs. Woffington Interspersed with Several Theatrical Anecdotes*. London: J. Swan, 1760.

Actor training from 1612 to 1727

There are several books on actors and acting from this period. The first is Thomas Heywood's Apology for Actors in 1612. Heywood seeks to justify acting as an art form, claiming its antiquity, dignity and the educational value of theatre performances. The second is John Bulwer's Chirologia and Chironomia of 1644, which details how hand gestures in daily life are to be understood and offers a description of gestures to be used in public speaking. The third is the Roscius Anglicanus, by John Downes 1708, which lists actors and companies of the day, including some lists of roles played by such actors. John Downes was the bookkeeper and prompter to Betterton's company. The fourth work, The Life of Mr Thomas Betterton, the Late Eminent Tragedian, with instructions how to use gesture, stance, facial expression and voice (Gildon) was written in 1710, and, finally, a fifth manual was written by Jesuit priest Franziskus Lang, Dissertatio de Actione Scenica, in 1727. This last work details stance, gesture and vocal technique in performance and was aimed at schoolboys learning to act gracefully.

John Bulwer's Chirologia

John Bulwer, baptized 1606, buried 1656, was a philosopher and medical doctor interested in human behaviour and gesture. In 1644, he wrote a slim volume called Chirologia, or the Natural

Language of the Hand. The book was aimed at public speakers, not necessarily the theatre stage, but nonetheless provides some insight into conventionalized hand gestures of the time, 'the Hand, that busy instrument is most talkative, whole language is as easily perceived and understood as if Man had another fountain of discourse in his Hand' (Bulwer 1). Bulwer claims that the hand is a substitute for the tongue and can represent all aspects of inner emotion and thought, 'It may well be called the tongue and general language of Human Nature' (Bulwer 3). He believed a hand can represent a whole dictionary of ideas:

For with our Hands,

we sue, intreat, beseech, solicit, call, allure, entice, dismiss, grant, deny, reprove, are supplicant, fear, threaten, abhor, repent, pray, trust, witness, accuse, declare our silence, condemn, absolve, show our astonishment, proffer, refuse, respect, give honour, adore, worship, despise, prohibit, reject, challenge, bargain, bow, swear, imprecate, humour, allow, give warning, command, reconcile, submit, defy, affront, offer injury, complement, argue, dispute, explode, confute, exhort, admonish, affirm, distinguish, urge, doubt, reproach, mock, approbe, dislike, encourage, recommend, flatter, applaud, exalt, humble, insult, adjure, confess, cherish, demand, crave, covet, bless, number, prove, confirm, salute, congratulate, entertain, give thanks, welcome, bid farewell, chide, bawl, consent, upbraid, envy, reward, offer force, pacify, condemn, disdain, disallow, forgive, offer peace, promise, perform, reply, invoke, request, repel, charge, deprecate, lament, condole, brag, boast, warrant, assure, enquire, direct, adopt, rejoice, show gladness, complain, despair, grieve, are sad and sorrowful, cry out, bewail, forbid, discomfort, ask, are angry, wonder, admire, pity, assent, order, rebuke, savour, sighs, despair, disparage, are earnest, importunate, refer, put to compromise, plight our faith, make a league of friendship, strike one good luck, take earnest, barter, exchange, show our agreement, express our liberality, show our benevolence, are illiberal, ask mercy, exhibit grace, show our displeasure, fret, chafe, fume, rage, revenge, crave audience, call for silence, prepare for an apology, give liberty of speech, take notice, warn one to forbear, keep off and be gone; take acquaintance, confess ourselves deceived by a mistake, make remonstrance of another's error, weep, give a pledge of aid, comfort, relieve, demonstrate, persuade, revolve, speak to, appeal, profess a willingness to strike, shew ourselves convinced, say we know somewhat which we will not tell, present a check to, silence, promise secrets, protest our innocence, manifest our love, enmity, hate and delight, provoke, hyperbolically extoll, enlarge our mirth with jollity and triumphant acclamations of delight, note and signify another's actions, the manner, place and time, as how, where, when, etc. (Bulwer 8–10)

Arms akimbo and 'camp'

Sometimes, a favoured gesture or hand movement can become an object of mockery. What was once a positive gesture is turned into a very negative one. This happened with the 'hands on hips' gesture. Originally, hands on hips 'arms akimbo' (in a keen bow) was used in portraiture of the aristocracy and military to show 'authority, pride of place . . . and manly valour' (King 55). It was used in the European court to reassert the sense of hierarchy and traditional authority of power (the restoration of the 'rightful' monarch; King 56). Inigo Jones's costume sketches for James I and Charles I show them both standing arms akimbo (King 56). Indeed, the further the elbows were extended from the body, the greater the amount of power: 'the Arm extended and lifted up signifies the Power of doing and accomplishing something; and it is the gesture of Authority, Vigour and Victory. . . . On the contrary, holding your Arms close is a sign of Bashfulness, Modesty and Diffidence' (King 244). Thus, standing with arms wide akimbo represented power – which does not necessarily mean 'manliness', however.

Later, 'arms akimbo' was mocked and scorned as 'just show'. Later still, it became a gesture of femininity because it seemed over-exaggerated, artificial, superficial, affected, 'Then with long strides advancing a few Paces, his left Hand settled upon his Hip, in a beautiful Bend, like that of the Handle of an old fashion'd Caudle-Cup, his Right remained immoveable across his manly Breast 'till numbness called its Partner to supply the Place; when, it relieved itself in the Position of the other Handle to the Caudle-Cup' (King 48). By the mid-1700s, Henry Mossop was mockingly nicknamed 'the tea pot actor' (King 48). Thus, conventional theatre gestures can be exaggerated and exploited for the sake of comedy and mocking. Susan Sontag suggests that the fashion for clear outward signs of status and gender in the 1600–1700s turned to mockery in the 1800s. Since then, 'actions and behaviour of utmost affectation, artificiality and flamboyance' (King 51) have become known as 'camp' which, in

Excavation One – the language of the hand

Review the list of words Bulwer thinks can be communicated with the hand alone. Working in pairs, each choose one word and create a hand gesture that captures it. See if your partner can identify the meaning. Continue for a few rounds.

Bulwer provides some illustrations of the gestures of the hand in daily life. These are in the section titled Chirologia, which simply describes hand gestures. First, there are several things that must *not* be done with the hands:

It is forbidden:

To snap the fingers.

To give secret messages by secret hand signals.

To stretch out the hands in length to a racked extent, or to erect them upward to their utmost elevation, or by a repeated gesture beyond the left shoulder so to throw back the hands that it is scarce safe for any man to remain behind them, to thrust out the arm, so that the side is openly discovered or to draw sinister circles or rashly fling up the hand . . .

To use the action of one that saws or cuts . . .

To represent a physician feeling the pulse of the arteries . . . or to show a lutenist striking the chords of an instrument.

Erect a finger to utmost extension.

To bring the fingers' ends to the breast, the hand hollow when we speak to ourselves, for this is unbecoming. (Bulwer 218)

Arms akimbo and to rest the turned-in back of the hand upon the side is an action of pride and ostentation.

No clapping.

No elbows out.

No scratching. (Bulwer 219)

Excavation Two – the forbidden hand

In pairs, review the list of forbidden actions of social interactions above. Have these changed over time? What other actions of the hand might you add to the list today?

Excavation Three - the everyday hand

Figures 4.1 and 4.2 show gestures of the everyday hand and their meanings. In pairs, create a similar table of ten of your own everyday hand gestures and their meanings. Remember, these must be universally understood and uphold social morals and manners.

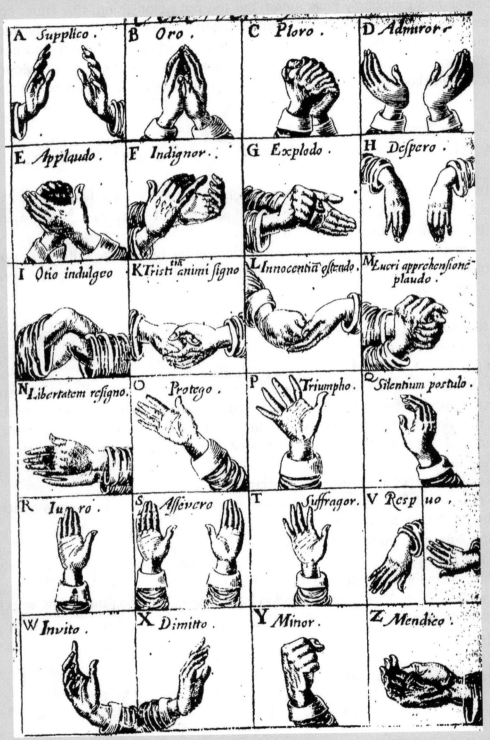

Figure 4.1 Everyday hand gestures from Bulwer's Chirologia I (Bulwer 115) © British Library Board (959.a.14). Images published with permission of ProQuest. Further reproduction is prohibited without permission.

A I entreat; B I pray; C I weep; D I admire; E I applaud; F I am indignant; G I explode in anger; H I despair; I I indulge in ease; K I show mental anguish; L I show innocence; M I applaud the taking of money; N I resign my liberty; O I protect; P I triumph; Q I demand silence; R I swear; S With steady faith, I call God to witness; T I permit; V I reject; W I invite; X I dismiss; Y I threaten; Z I beg.

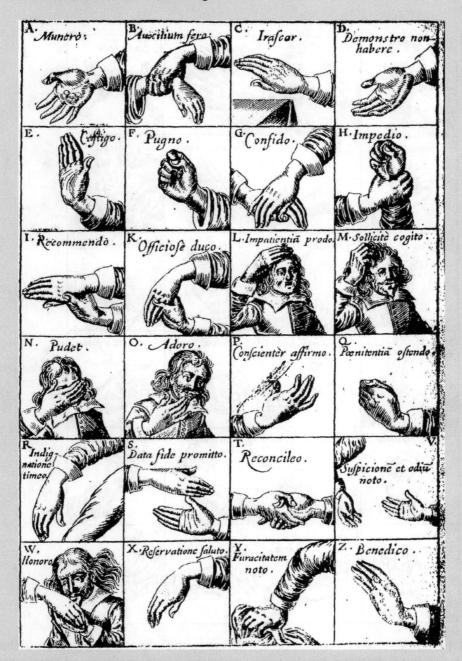

Figure 4.2 Everyday hand gestures from Bulwer's Chirologia II (Bulwer 117) © British Library Board (959.a.14). Images published with permission of ProQuest. Further reproduction is prohibited without permission.

A I reward; B I bring aid; C I am angry; D I show I do not have; E I chastise; F I fight; G I trust; H I hinder; I I recommend; K I lead in an official capacity; L I show impatience; M I am worried; N I am ashamed; O I appeal to; P I conscientiously assert; Q I show contrition; R I am afraid and indignant; S I pledge my faith; T I reconcile; V I note suspicion and hatred; W I honour; X I greet with reservation; Y I show thievery; Z I bless.

Survey the terrain

Is the language of the hand free of race, gender, ethnicity, age, social standing?

The second section of Bulwer's book, the Chironomia, prescribes what gestures should be used in public performance. Figures 4.3–4.5 show illustrations of the gestures and their meanings.

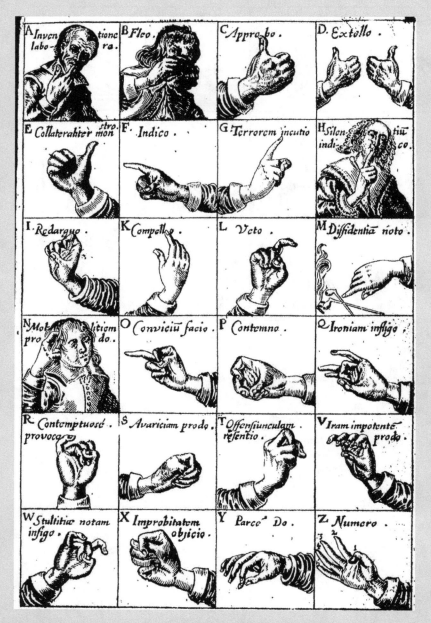

Figure 4.3 Hand gestures for public performance from Bulwer's Chironomia I (Bulwer 143) © British Library Board (959.a.14). Images published with permission of ProQuest. Further reproduction is prohibited without permission.

A I work in discovery; B I weep; C I approve; D I extol; E I show both sides of an issue; F I point; G I inflict terror; H I indicate silence; I I refute; K I summon; L I disapprove; M I show hesitancy; N I betray weakness; O I provoke an argument; P I condemn; Q I impose irony; R I provoke contemptuously; S I present greed; T I resent a small offense; V I betray a mild anger; W I make the sign of foolishness; X I accuse of improbability; Y I give sparingly; Z I count.

A to call for silence; **B** in one's humble opinion; **C** to ask the audience to listen; **D** to gesture with benevolence; **E** to prepare to speak; **F** to show admiration, **G** to exhort, cheer, embolden and encourage; **H** to show the reason for something; **I** to contradict oneself for the sake of argument; **K** to be moved with sudden indignation and to be amazed with fear; **L** to refer to oneself; **M** to refuse, abhor, detest, abominate or repel; **N** to clarify; **O** to congratulate, exclaim, a sign of joy; **P** to show antithesis or opposite arguments; **Q** to number the arguments; **R** to show kindness or benevolence; **S** to show pity; **T** to show something vast in size; **V** to turn away in disgust; **W** to despise, to detest; **X** to invoke, doubt, accuse; **Y** to show grief and sorrow; **Z** to dismiss with a blessing.

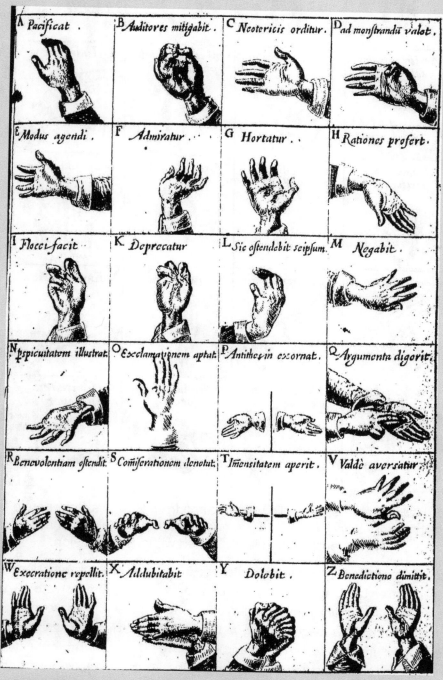

Figure 4.4 Hand gestures for public performance from Bulwer's Chironomia II (Bulwer 193) © British Library Board (959.a.14). Images published with permission of ProQuest. Further reproduction is prohibited without permission.

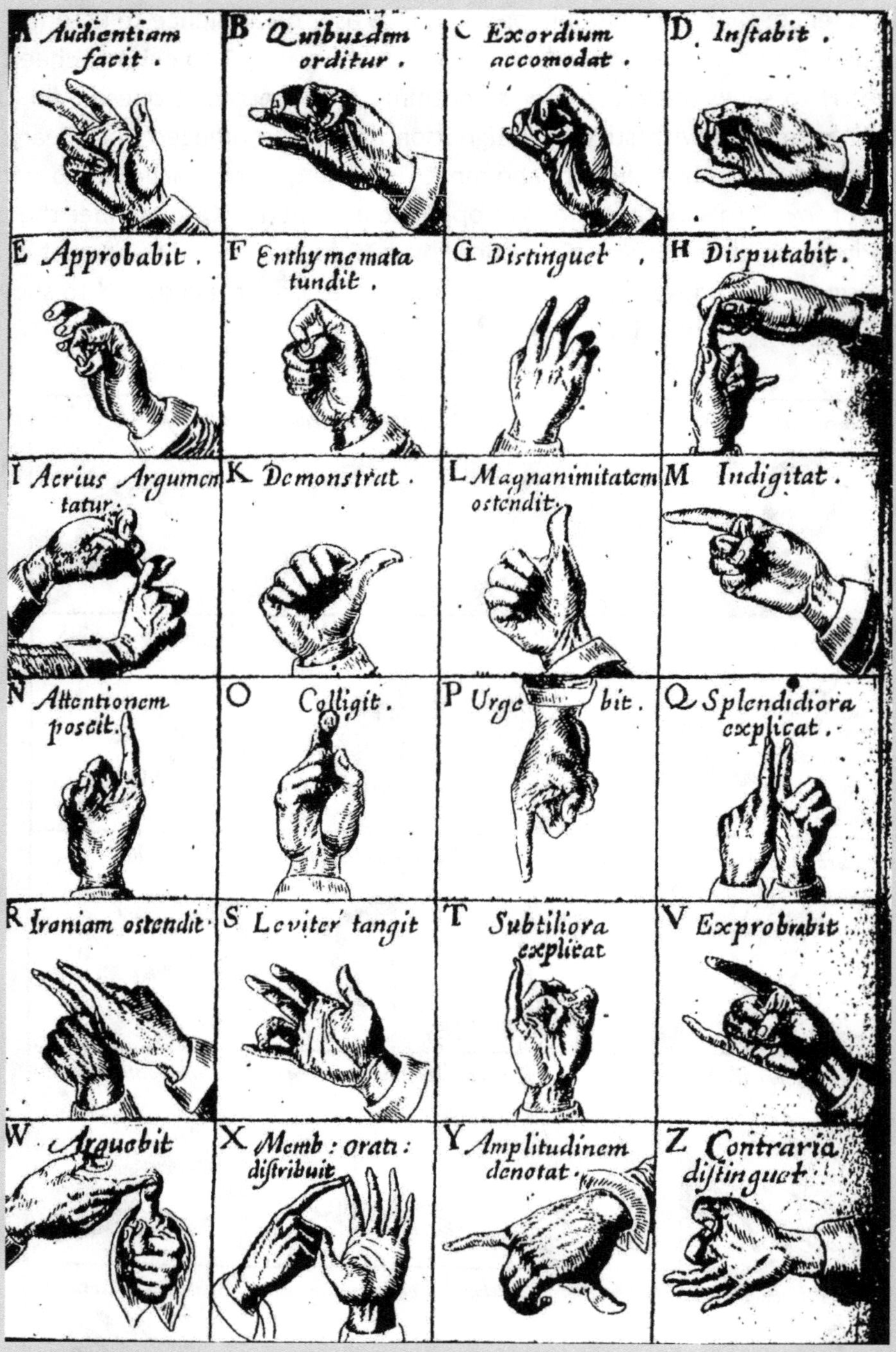

Figure 4.5 Hand gestures for public performance from Bulwer's Chironomia III (Bulwer 213) © British Library Board (959.a.14). Images published with permission of ProQuest. Further reproduction is prohibited without permission.

A to demand silence and procure an audience; B to begin the introduction; C to make a preface; D to insist or urge; E to distinguish or approve; F to demonstrate; G to count out two or three chief points to an ignorant multitude; H to dispute; I to argue more vehemently; K to demonstrate; L to show magnanimity; M to show indignation with great emphasis; N to demand attention, if moved, to threaten and denounce; O to confirm, collect, refute; P to urge; Q to exalt the force that flows from more splendid and glorious elocution; R to show ironical intention; S to handle a matter lightly; T to explain more subtle things; V to reproach; W to be insistent; X to number the arguments; Y to emphasize; Z to show contraries.

Excavation Four – Desdemona's hands

In pairs, take the text of Desdemona and Othello Act 5 Scene II, and choose appropriate gestures from those illustrated above to interpret the scene. First, try this with no spoken dialogue, then with speech added.

Setting the compass

If the language of the hands is gender-neutral, is spoken text also gender-neutral?

turn, suggested homosexuality. Sontag explains that with the restoration of the monarchy came a desire for a sense of élite, unnatural, artificial, highly over-exaggerated, 'specialness' that might be defined as camp. These are just codes – ways of behaving used by everyone in order to 'fit in'. However, the artificiality or affectation and flamboyance encompassed in the word 'camp' is now seen in all walks of life from Instagram to the music world and is not automatically linked to homosexuality any more.

Thomas Betterton's rules

Thomas Betterton (1635–1710), actor and theatre manager, played the male roles to Kynaston's female roles. His biographer claims that he felt young actors did nothing but get drunk and never turn up for rehearsals, when in fact, 'Action indeed has a natural excellence in it, superior to all other qualities; action is motion and motion is the support of nature, which without it would again sink into the sluggish mass of chaos' (Gildon 26). Gildon is writing about Mr Betterton's advice on acting. It is the first attempt at a 'system' of acting and yet seems highly contemporary. Betterton's thoughts about the language of theatre are not dissimilar to Bulwer's. He begins:

> I shall therefore begin with the government, order and balance as I may say of the whole body, and thence I shall proceed to the regiment and proper motions of the head, the eyes, the eyebrows and indeed the whole face, and I shall conclude with the actions of the hands, more copious and various than all other parts of the body. (Gildon 57)

Mr Betterton gives some general rules regarding the actions of the hands:

> When you speak of yourself the right, not the left hand must be applied to the bosom, declaring you own faculties and passions, your heart, your soul, or your conscience. (Gildon 75)
>
> You must be sure as you begin your action with what you say, so you must end it when you have done speaking. (Gildon 75)
>
> In the lifting up the hands to preserve the Grace, you ought not to raise them above the eyes; to stretch them farther might disorder and distort the body; nor must it be very little lower, because that position gives a beauty to the figure. (Gildon 77)
>
> You must never let either of your hands hang down as if lame or dead; for that is very disagreeable to the eye and argues no passion in the imagination. In short, your hands must always be in view of your eyes and so corresponding with the motions of the head, eyes and body that the spectator may see their concurrence, everyone in its own way to

signify the same thing, which will make a more agreeable and by consequence a deeper impression on their senses and understanding. (Gildon 77)

Of the body, Mr Betterton advises:

The place and posture of the body ought not to be changed every moment, since so fickle an agitation is trifling and light: nor, on the other hand, should it always keep the same position, fixt like a pillar or marble statue. (Gildon 57)

Excavation Five – graceless hands

Review the list of 'not to's in Bulwer's Chirologia and Mr Betterton's advice. In groups of four to five, create a comic scene in 2 minutes that deliberately uses all the 'wrong' sorts of gesture and movement on stage. Compare to the concept of grace explained in Chapter 5.

Whole-class reckoning

Discuss the 'rights' and 'wrongs' of action on stage and intention in performance.

Franziskus Lang, Jesuit priest and drama teacher

While in England the choristers of prestigious schools focused on the classics were engaged in performing and entertaining at court, on the Continent, regular performances were held in and by schools as a vital aspect of the curriculum, particularly in Jesuit schools, and especially in conservative Austria and Bavaria. Although the Jesuit priest Franziskus Lang's work was not published until 1727, could Betterton have seen a copy? Thomas Betterton claims to have seen a manuscript by a Jesuit 'who wrote on this subject' (Gildon 43). The Jesuits are a religious order of the Catholic church focused on education and missionary work. It was thought that by performing plays, the boys would learn not only how to structure a powerful thought in speech but also improve their Latin and, at the same time, be educated in the moral of the story being played. Since girls were not permitted to attend these schools, the boys were obliged to play all the roles in the chosen drama. The Jesuit priest, Franziskus Lang, wrote *Dissertatio de Actionae Scenica* specifically for these student actors. What all these works show is that the rules of public performance, gesture and stance of the 1600s–1700s were heavily conventionalized or fixed. Lang wrote that he had been trained as a child in the art of speaking, but 'little about the body' (F. Lang 158). Thus, his book is an attempt to redress that situation. 'Through correct performance, the actor can incite pure and useful emotions in the spectators'.

Franziskus Lang (1654) was born in Bavaria, now Germany. From the age of 10 he attended Jesuit school and performed there before becoming a priest in 1671 and teaching grammar, rhetoric, poetry and drama (F. Lang 312). Lang was a key figure in Jesuit theatre in Munich and surroundings and wrote his book for training actors, *Dissertatio de Actione Scenica* in 1727. Lang's information was derived from classical Roman sources reflecting the passion of this era for the ancient classics of Greece and Rome. It emphasizes, once again, that intercultural and historical research so often feeds creative innovation in theatre. Here is his advice for the budding actor (F. Lang 161).

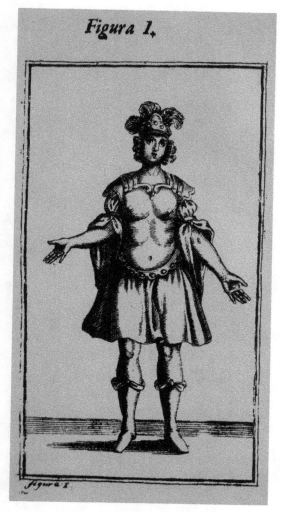

Figure 4.6 On entering the stage (F. Lang 40–41) Bayerische Staatsbibliothek München, Res/L. eleg.g.222 Figura I.

On entering the stage (Figure 4.6)

'The most important task of the actor on entering the stage is to show the stance and facial expression of the character being played directly to the spectators so that they can immediately read the mood of that character' (F. Lang 189). Lang felt that 'the actions come before the words to give the spectator time to know what will be said' (F. Lang 195) and 'when speech has finished, the emotion must be held a little longer, rather than just dropped at once' (F. Lang 196). 'Always keep the correct position on stage and the eyes are always turned towards the audience' (see Figure 4.7).

On walking

'When the sole of the foot is placed on the floor, the first thing to notice is that it must never point in the same direction as its partner, but each foot is noticeably distanced from the previous one as it is placed on the boards, and so that the toes of the one foot point in one direction and those of the other point in another direction. The stance is always at an angle to the audience, sometimes less' (F. Lang 171).

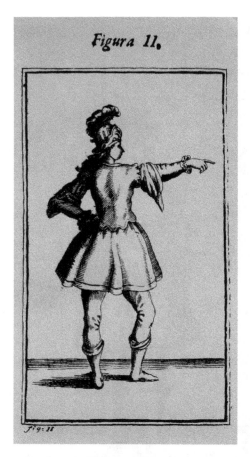

Figure 4.7 Eyes always turn to the audience (F. Lang 54–55) Bayerische Staatsbibliothek München, Res/L.eleg.g.222 Figura II.

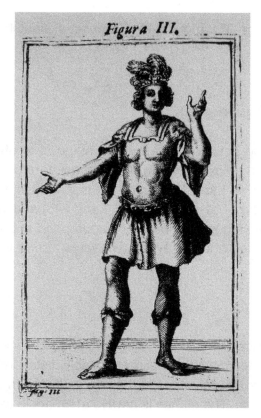

Figure 4.8 On walking and pausing (F. Lang 18–19) Bayerische Staatsbibliothek München, Res/L.eleg.g.222 Figura III.

'The stage walk must be completed in three to four steps and the 45 degree angle between the feet must be maintained. If the actor desires to move from one spot to another, and thus step forwards, it will be inappropriate if he simply moves from the static position without first drawing the foot that was in front of the other backwards in the opposite direction. Thus, the foot that was originally in front is drawn back and then moved forward but further forward than it was before. Now the second foot may follow and be placed in front of the first foot: but the first foot, cannot remain where it is, but moves in front of the second . . . all along while the feet are set down diagonally from each other. First make steps 1,2,3,4 and then make a slight pause' (see Figure 4.8).

'When turning from one side to the other, the feet remain in the position of the Crux Scenica (dramatic cross) and the body stays open to the audience, at an angle' (see Figure 4.9).

'Of course, care must be taken if there are others on the stage. Then the steps have to be smaller and not disturb the other players or get in their way' (F. Lang 175).

Sometimes, lines were drawn with charcoal and chalk on the stage to show the apprentices how to walk across it, because it is not natural and has to be learnt and practised. 'Knees are always bent. . . . In order to achieve this, the actor's back leg and thigh needs to rise at the hip on the corresponding side so that the slightly tilted body rest entirely on the back leg and hip' (see Figure 4.10).

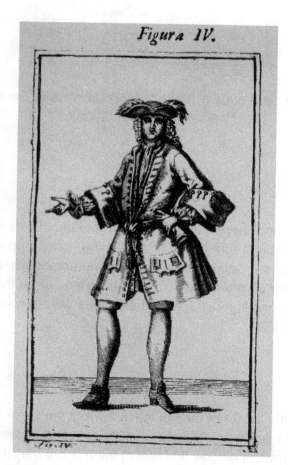

Figure 4.9 The crux scenica (F. Lang 42–43) Bayerische Staatsbibliothek München, Res/L.eleg.g.222 Figura IV.

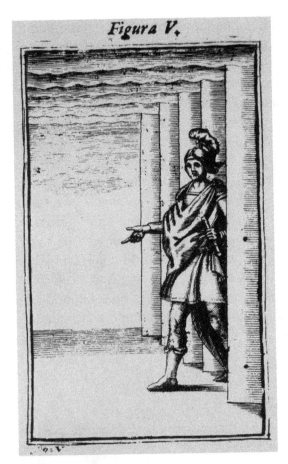

Figure 4.10 The slightly tilted body (F. Lang 26–27) Bayerische Staatsbibliothek München, Res/L.eleg.g.222 Figura V.

On hips

'The hips are the seat of all movement, and bending at the hip affects the entire torso according to the needs of the play, through turning in, straightening, pulling up or twisting of the hips for the different requirements of the performance so that different expressive poses are created . . . hip movements must also be co-ordinated with the shoulders, since these parts of the body are interrelated so that as soon one is moved, the other moves with it, in order to present a pleasing shape in the body' (F. Lang 177).

On arm positions

'The play of hands and arms must not take place in front of the body nor may they occur below the level of the belt' (see Figure 4.11). 'Hands must never be stretched out on either side in the same formation, nor may arms or elbows find rest at the hip, nor may the fingers be stretched out straight when the hand is extended' (F. Lang 171).

'On stage, keep the arms freely away from the body rather than keeping them closely to the hips or sides. . . when the two arms are outstretched, never do this the same on both sides, one can be higher, the other lower, one straight, the other bent' (F. Lang 179).

'Especially shy actors or young ones, like to keep their hands in their pockets, but this is clumsy and ugly' (F. Lang 179).

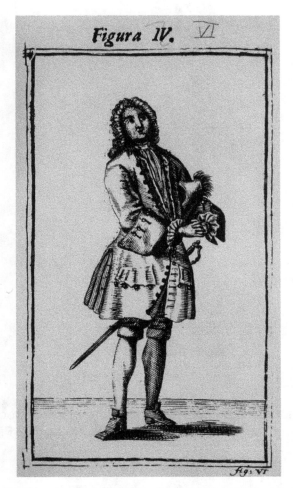

Figure 4.11 Gestures must not be made in front of the body (F. Lang 50–51) Bayerische Staatsbibliothek München, Res/L.eleg.g.222 Figura VI.

'Do not allow the arms to hang straight down, or shoot straight up like bullets . . . sometimes the right hand might stretch out but not to its full length unless pointing, while the left arm might be in the shape of a handle to the side' (F. Lang 180).

'Wrists should be flexible . . . the index finger is stretched out straight and the other fingers are gradually bent towards the open palm, but the fingers should not be held as if they were made of wood or were too stiff to move' (see Figure 4.12).

'Different hand positions can be made by more or less extreme bending in, stretching out . . . and I must stress that the utmost effort is required for hand exercises, long and diligent hard work if the fingers are to fulfil their task aesthetically, and execute those gestures that individually belong to the role and always appear graceful in movement' (F. Lang 181).

'Some people like to wear gloves, but I have never seen this or heard about it before and I do not think it is a good idea. . . . Since the hand is the most perfect tool of performance art, it must remain uncovered, so that all those present can witness such movements as are dictated by Nature and Art and be open to be moved by them' (F. Lang 182; see Figure 4.13).

'A gesture is mostly undertaken with the right hand which means the left hand has to support it. A good actor touches his breast when talking about himself or at least points to it' (F. Lang 184).

'Do not raise the hands above the eyes to block sight of the eyes and do not hide the hands in the chest or pockets. Hands should never be balled into fists – only if the character being represented is a peasant, or the rage is very violent, can fists be shown' (F. Lang 185).

'Never raise a sound by clapping hands together unless in a comedy when laughing about someone or mocking them' and 'never snap the fingers to call someone' (F. Lang 185).

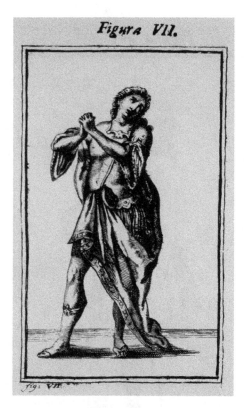

Figure 4.12 Fingers should not be held as if they were made of wood (F. Lang 28–29) Bayerische Staatsbibliothek München, Res/L.eleg.g.222 Figura VII.

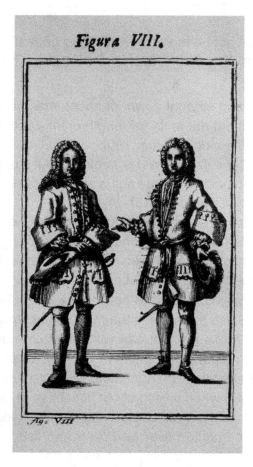

Figure 4.13 Do not wear gloves Bayerische Staatsbibliothek München, Res/L.eleg.g.222 Figura VIII.

On gesture

'Gesture must not be used as it is in real life, or as mime: for example, chopping wood, shooting an arrow, hitting something with a stick, digging in the earth, throwing a ball and various other kinds of similar activity. These are to be indicated rather than carried out realistically' (F. Lang 185–186).

The ten key positions of acting prescribed by Lang

1. We show admiration by raising both hands towards the upper chest, while the palms are facing the audience.

2. We show disdain with a face turned to the left, stretching out the slightly raised hands in order to push the distasteful object away to the opposite side. We can do the same action with the right hand alone, where the hand is slightly bent towards the wrist and at the same time fearfully drive away the object of distaste with repeated movements.

3. We implore by raising both hands, palms facing inward, or lowering the same, or with palms together and interlocking fingers.

4. We show suffering and grief by interlocking the hands like a comb and either raising them to the chest or lowering them towards the belt. The same emotion can be shown with one slightly outstretched arm, and the right hand turned towards the chest.

5. We cry out by having arms stretched up in a becoming way, both hands are somewhat spread out and turned to each other, can also be somewhat bent outwards, whereby the meaning of the emotion can be presented.

6. We accuse someone by bending in three fingers and stretching out the index finger, or with a bent middle finger and the other three stretched out, or with simply with a bent middle finger.

7. We show encouragement with arms and hands somewhat open and turned towards the person we are encouraging, as if we intended to embrace them.

8. We show questioning by raising the slightly upturned hand.

9. We show regret with a closed fist against the chest.

10. We show fear by pressing the right hand to the chest whereby the first four fingers are drawn into a point; the hand should then be lowered and left to hang down at the side of the body.

(F. Lang 186–187)

Excavation Six – the learning play

The Jesuits were adamant that in learning to act in a play, young people would learn about morals and about correct human behaviour. That is, acting was a learning opportunity for the actor, not just the audience. This same idea was taken up by Bertolt Brecht in Germany in the 1920s and early 1930s, when he wrote a series of Lehrstücke or 'learning plays' for young people.

In class, read the two plays, He Who Says Yes and He Who Says No, which Brecht adapted from the Japanese No play Taniko. They are barely four pages each. The play deals with conformity, consent, group and individual thought and taking action.

After reading through, as a class, think-pair-share-reflect on what you have just read. Those who think the boy should go, the Yes Sayers, move to the right of the studio. The No Sayers move to the left.

Pay attention to the Epic theatre devices Brecht uses such as narration, chorus, roles defined by social roles and not names (teacher, students), scenes played onstage at the same time though separate in time and space, use of verse, repetition of action and dialogue, self-narration, lack of scenery, a moral dilemma reflecting society's inhumanity and so on. As a whole-class exercise, try roughly walking through the two plays one after the other (which goes first?) still holding scripts.

Make another foot survey after the read through – Yes Sayers to the right, No Sayers to the left. Has there been a change?

Setting the compass

Acting is more than 'pretending'; it is also taking action. The importance of learning to act in developing understanding of the self and the world.

Excavation Seven – believability

The idea that the body can communicate in its own 'language' just like spoken language is a key aspect of modern actor training and behavioural science. It is even applied to police interrogation techniques. What Every Body Is Saying (Navarro), written by a former FBI agent of interrogation, identifies aspects of human behaviour that reveal whether or not someone is telling the truth (or acting); whether someone is feeling confident or not – in fact, all sorts of clues about how a person might be feeling are revealed in the way they move (or don't move) their bodies.

'Non-verbal behaviour or body language is a means of transmitting information . . . except it is achieved through facial expressions, gestures, touching (haptics), physical movements (kinesics), posture, body adornment – clothes, jewellery, hairstyle, etc.' (Navarro 3–4). He calls these nonverbal behaviours 'tells' like in a poker game. These reveals or tells cannot be determined until a baseline behaviour has been identified and the context of the situation taken into account. Baseline simply means the kinds of actions someone does all the time. As an observer of nonverbal cues, one must look out for sudden or unexpected changes in behaviour. Second, the nonverbal cue happens within a particular situation or context. Feet hopping up and down might be joyous feet, impatient feet or angry feet, so the context of situation will help interpretation.

Look at some of the nonverbal behaviours from Navarro's book listed below and practise them with a partner. Let your partner critique you whether your 'tell' was convincingly natural or 'put on'.

Feet

'Feet are the most important location of honesty since one can control the facial expression, but not often what the feet are doing. Never interview a criminal when their feet are under the table' (Navarro 53; see Table 4.12).

Table 4.12 Foot positions (Navarro 53)

Note the way the feet are pointing towards the person or object = interest; away from the person or object = wanting to run.	Feet wide apart = struggling to take command again by taking up as much space as possible.	Standing with legs crossed = feeling comfortable with company since balance is reduced and the person feels safe despite this.

Feet mirroring the dialogue partner = a sign of comfort and confidence.	Standing with one foot pointing towards the door = wanting to leave.	Gravity-defying feet that bounce, rock, jiggle = positive feelings.

Torso

'The torso is an area that houses vital internal organs, so the brain seeks to protect it when threatened or challenged' (Navarro 85; see Table 4.13).

Shoulders and arms

Arms are there to protect us and 'can be counted on to reveal true sentiments or intentions' (Navarro 109; see Table 4.14).

Table 4.13 Torso positions (Navarro 85)

Leaning in towards someone or something = interest, admiration, confidence.	Facing the object or person showing the vulnerable front torso as to a small child = confidence, comfort.	Torso shielding with folded arms, buttoning a jacket, holding schoolbooks in front of the chest, using arms across the body to examine a watch, straighten a tie = protection of vulnerable person.
Leaning away from someone or something = fear, disgust, disinterest.	Torso embellishment – drawing attention to torso through letter jacket, official badge, lanyard = confidence and authority.	Torso splay – spreading the body in seated position like a bored teenager = adopting position of authority, disrespecting everyone else.

Table 4.14 Shoulders and arms (Navarro 109)

Both shoulders in a shrug = authentic 'I don't know'.	Arms that defy gravity usually = happy, confident, positive feelings.	Arms behind the back = high status and don't touch me.
One shoulder in a shrug, or partial shrug = lack of commitment to the statement made.	Arms sinking or close to the body = negative feelings, withdrawal, injury, threat.	Arms and elbows on armrests indicate territorial struggle for higher status.
Arms akimbo = authority.	Hands behind the head = power and authority.	Stretched arms over the back of a chair = struggling for power.
Look out for adornments on arms, like expensive watches and jewellery.	Turtling: pulling the shoulders up high so the neck disappears = reaction to a negative event.	Breathing rapidly making the torso expand = stressed and ready for fight or flight.

Hands

'If you wish to enhance your effectiveness as a persuasive speaker – at home, at work, with your friends – attempt to become more expressive in your use of hand movements' (Navarro 134-135; see Table 4.15).

Table 4.15 Arms (Navarro 134–135)

To show trust, hands must always be visible; not kept under a table or in a pocket.	Touching the face, neck, necklace, earlobe when asked a difficult question is a movement of comfort to cover embarrassment and stay calm.	Sliding hands along the thighs when sitting to dry sweaty palms = anxiety and discomfort.
Steepling the hands = high confidence. Women steeple lower, men steeple at chest level.	Thumbs out of pockets while fingers are in = high confidence. Thumbs in pockets with hands out = low confidence.	Genital framing – thumbs inside waistband or pockets and fingers splayed, framing the genitals = high confidence.

Excavation Eight – the 'tell'

Now with the same partner, prepare three short sequences of 30 seconds of action, one to accompany each of 'two truths and a lie'. This means you will have to share two things that are true about you, and one which is made up. Can you hide the 'tell' and lie convincingly?

Change partners and perform your 'two truths and a lie'. Can your new partner see the 'tell'? How did they know? How were they deceived? Change places and repeat.

Change partners once more and repeat the exercise both ways.

Whole-class reckoning

Is actor training like learning to lie? The power of the body to communicate truths and lies. The language of the body can lie.

Resources, actor training

Bulwer, John. *Chirologia or the Natural Language of the Hand*. London: Thom. Harper and Henry Twyford, 1644. Images produced by ProQuest as part of Early English Books Online. www.proquest.com.
Downes, John. *Roscius Anglicanus*. Ed. Montague Summers. Robarts University of Toronto, 1928.
Heywood, Thomas. *Apology for Actors 1612*. London: Schoberl, 1841.
Gildon, Charles. *The Life of Mr. Thomas Betterton 1710*. New York: Augustus M. Kelly, 1970.
King, Thomas A. *The Gendering of Men 1600–1750, Vol. 2, Queer Articulations*. Madison: University of Wisconsin Press, 2008.
Lang, F. Dissertatio de actione scenica, cum figuris eandem explicantibus. Munich, 1727.
Lang, Franziskus. *Abhandlung über die Schauspielkunst trans and ed Alexander Rudlin*. Bern: Franke, 1975. English trans. of this section by Riley.
Navarro, Joe. *What Every Body is Saying*. New York: Harper, 2008.

CHAPTER 5

With gender – world theatre

The lost boy. I grew up in a huge, sprawling family where undivided gardens allowed for children from the street to meet and play with no boundaries. Every summer a child from the Italian orphanage and various foster children arrived to stay; our friends also came to play and stayed over for days on end. All the gardens backed onto a large field, sometimes planted with wheat, sometimes left to fallow; a tiny trodden footpath crossed it diagonally towards a disused canal that flowed towards narrow tributaries with bridges and locks. What a space to play! Because the siblings were all girls but one; the father of the family often absent for work and substitute nannies and au-pairs also female, it was thought a wise idea to remove the boy child and place him in a more 'male' environment. My brother was sent away to a boys' boarding school. The loss of my brother weighed very heavily on me. Even when he came home for the holidays, things were never the same again. I was sent to an all-girl's school – my world became even narrower. Houses were built on the field.

A decade later, in China, my theatre Master suggested I perform a piece with him on stage. He would enact the painted-face character of a hearty, life-loving monk who escapes the monastery to taste the joys of wine. I would play the part of a youth travelling the countryside with a yoke over my shoulders bearing wine to sell. He taught me each line; each movement, stance and walk; each gesture, facial expression, song; and a comic fight where I battle with the drunken monk to prevent him getting hold of more wine and drinking it without paying me. He costumed me in loose silk trousers, a jacket, a neck scarf and a little hat; he painted my face as a young boy with red lips and a rose pink shade over the eyes, lifting the outer corners of each eyebrow with a cord tied around my head to give the impression that my eyes slanted boyishly upwards at sharp angle.

The difficult thing about performing Chinese theatre is that the performer dictates the rhythm and pace of the singing and movement. The musicians follow the performer with their eyes, never once looking at their instruments. They play what rhythm they see. So, I had to enter with great buoyant strides, singing, swinging the poles with their heavy wine jars on my shoulders, calling

DOI: 10.4324/9781003080800-6

'wine for sale!' and stop suddenly when I spotted the monk. I was the initiator, the activator, of the scene and its pace; my role was the active, cheeky, impoverished, but cheerful foil to the great monk. I tasted what it might feel like to be a boy.

No theatre

There are two ways of transcribing this traditional Japanese theatre form: No and Noh. Both refer to a Japanese character that means 'special skill, or ability'. The No theatre is a masked theatre developed from songs and dances from the 14th century in Japan. Originally played by Buddhist priests, it is performed in a temple complex on a roofed and raised square stage, open on three sides with an entrance bridge stage right. The architecture and geomantic orientation of the stage is significant; modern No theatres replicate this temple-like structure. The actors are always male, and the tradition is passed down through families from father to son, nephew and grandson. A No performance can last all day: five plays in a row with comic relief from its counterpart, Kyogen, in between. Musicians and a chorus, singing to accompany movement, or to reflect the main actor's feelings, are always present onstage. The masks are made of wood and are smaller than the performer's face. The mask is kept in a special pouch, and when removing the mask from the pouch before the performance, the actor treats the mask as if it were a real person. The tilting and angling of the mask can significantly affect its expression (see Chapter 3). There is no set and very few props. The repertoire consists of ancient tales of real and fictional events including dreams, ghost plays and plays about mythical beings and visions. There are no lighting effects since the form derived from outdoor theatre. The goal of a No performance was to 'pacify, pleasure and move' the audience, according to Zeami, the great No actor and theorist.

Performers

Boys are trained in No theatre from about the age of 7 in apprenticeship to older actors. Often, the children live with the actor in his house for a period of learning if the child is not already a direct member of the family. The master instructs the pupil in basic movement patterns, voice, stance and gesture. Learning by watching and imitating is key. An adolescent student will also learn all the backstage tasks such as folding, packing and looking after costumes, making props and preparing for transporting them between theatres as well as maintaining respectful relations with everyone who works in the theatre on and off stage. Actors are said to emerge in their early 20s, peak in their early 30s, decline in their early 40s. Within seven strictly observed stages of training, all students will learn the three different types of role: aged style (rotai), feminine style (nyotai) and the martial style (guntai).

Audience

The No audience is silent and sometimes spectators read the play text along with the play. No theatre started out as a popular entertainment among the lower classes and was performed at temple festivals. Since the 1800s, however, the audience was increasingly made up of the educated and the elite; now, tickets are costly and No requires a level of spiritual and scholarly awareness. Attending a performance is also meditative as it has religious and philosophical content: the contemplation of the events on stage may bring the spectator closer to achieving nirvana or a state of perfection.

Excavation One – moulding a sequence – kata

The movements in No are made up of dance patterns named kata, which means *mould* or *form*, like the mould one might pour liquid bronze into. The kata are fixed dance sequences, and they are always performed in the same way, as they have become conventions (rules) of No. Each play consists of predetermined kata sequences which are also fixed and unchanging. There are no more than about 30 kata in No theatre in total. These are the 'ground patterns' around which a particular movement is based, and they can be performed with an open or closed fan (Bethe and Brazell 27).

Make your own kata:

Stand in a space with eyes closed and write your name in the air with your finger.

Increase the size of your signature by using the whole hand.

Increase the size of your signature by using the entire arm.

Repeat several times until this movement is fixed.

Now, still with eyes closed, draw your signature using the entire arm and add some different levels – crouching, stretching, bending and so on.

Repeat several times until this movement is fixed.

Now, still with eyes closed, draw your signature with the entire arm, different levels and add a turning in a full-360 circular movement on the spot as if you were a weathervane. Keep the movement fluid and consider shifting levels as you turn.

Repeat several times until this movement is fixed.

Transfer this movement to the map of the Japanese No stage, starting at 1; now move your feet in an anticlockwise circle through all the numbers to end with a flourish at 9.

Repeat several times until this movement is fixed.

You have now created your own personal kata.

Excavation Two – symbolic topographies

Patterning of movement in space can offer another level of theatrical communication, by using space to convey a specific meaning. The No stage is divided numerically to show the movement of the actor from the entrance to centre stage (see Figure 5.1). The actor always enters at 1, from the entrance bridge, and follows the numbers in an anticlockwise spiral to end in a magnificent pose at 9. The entrance on stage is usually a left-turning circle.

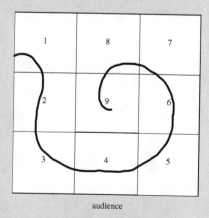

audience

Figure 5.1 The No stage is divided numerically.

The line of the actor's movement from 1 to 9 in a left-turning spiral describes the symbol of Yin and Yang (see Figure 5.2).

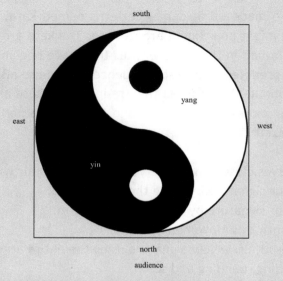

Figure 5.2 The No stage is divided by the yinyang symbol.

The balance of Yin and Yang is a philosophy of opposites held in harmony rather than conflict – there are elements of each in the other, and the flow of the line seeming to separate them is curved, fluid and inclusive. The elements represented are many, but include aspects for Yang, such as light, red, warmth, sun, energy, fire, male, and the Yin includes aspects such as dark, cloudy, cold, moon, passive, female. The Yinyang diagram expresses the idea that all these aspects are essential to each other where the whole is greater than the individual parts.

Each vertical division of the No stage is also given a value: the first column represents shin: formal, elaborate and complete; the middle column represents gyo: partially simplified, semiformal; and the third column represents so: simplified and informal (see Figure 5.3).

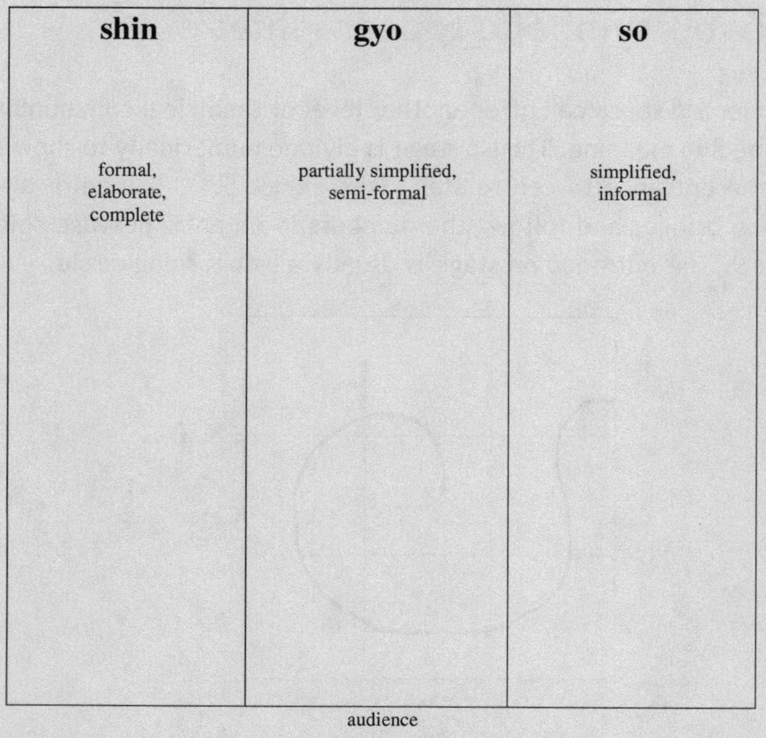

shin	gyo	so
formal, elaborate, complete	partially simplified, semi-formal	simplified, informal

audience

Figure 5.3 The No stage is divided vertically for formal aesthetics.

Combining the Yinyang value and the level of formality, each square of the stage contains two layers of meaning. When the actor moves from square to square, he is, in effect, bringing those aspects to life by his touch. For example, square 3, at downstage right, represents Yang suggesting active, bright, masculine as well as highly elaborate and formal, so a great deal of action on stage occurs here. Diagonally opposite square 7, at upstage left, on the other hand, represents Yin suggesting passive, cloudy, female as well as very simplified, informal, so little action happens here (Bethe and Brazell 20). A similar division of the stage based on a mathematical, magical formula is seen in traditional Chinese theatre (Riley 237).

Think, pair, share

Why are there such strict rules in Japanese No theatre? What do you think about the division of aspects into masculine and feminine? Are there such gender contrasts in other forms of theatre? Does this reflect gender differences in life?

Excavation Three – rhythmic topographies of jo-ha-kyu

The No stage is further divided into three horizontal rows which are given rhythmic values jo, ha and kyu roughly meaning: beginning – break – and rapid (see Figure 5.4). A movement should begin slowly, increase in speed, before stopping or pausing, and then rapidly come to an end. The cycle repeats itself ad infinitum.

Ann Bogart describes this pattern as introduction, exposition and denouement or resistance, rupture and acceleration; or hop, skip and jump (Bogart and Landau 147). Each No play has a jo-ha-kyu movement within it; each scene has jo-ha-kyu; each single movement has jo-ha-kyu. In 1920s Russia, Vsevolod Meyerhold devised a system of biomechanics that used a similar breakdown of stage action: otkas – a movement in the opposite direction to prepare; posyl, the action itself; and stoika, a definite stop bringing the movement to a close, but serving as a springboard for the next movement to begin, like jo-ha-kyu. The same pattern is also described in Commedia dell'arte performance as the actor draws back before moving forward, pulls to the left before moving off to the right, and this exists in traditional Chinese theatre too.

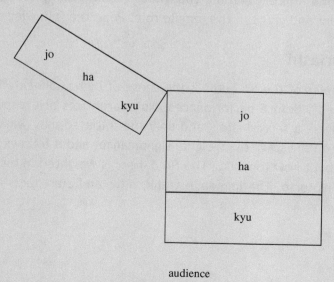

audience

Figure 5.4 The No stage is divided horizontally for jo-ha-kyu.

Add pace and rhythm to your kata sequence. Start in the jo area at square 1. Your kata sequence must begin at jo, which represents the first phase, 'when the force is put in motion as if overcoming a resistance'. Build in pace and speed towards ha, which is the 'the transition phase, rupture of the resistance, increase of the motion' before landing at square 3 representing kyu, the sudden stop, for a magnificent pose (mie) before continuing on to jo to start the cycle again.

Excavation Four – naming your stage

Using the kata sequence derived from your name or creating a new kata to represent some other aspect of your identity, design an appropriate symbolic mapping on the stage floor. Imprint your kata on squares, rows, columns, symbols of meaning that you have designed to represent aspects of yourself.

Whole-class reckoning

The significance of topography in communicating meaning.

A theatre performance can unify opposites. What relevance might this have for the concept of 'All the world's a playhouse'?

Try out Samuel Beckett's piece for four actors, Quad.

Excavation Five – the female role

In No theatre, there are three main kinds of role and all actors perform them. Actors do not specialize in one or the other. The three role types are: the aged rotai, the feminine jotai and martial guntai (Zeami). In this excavation, you will be focusing on either the walk – suriashi, or the concept of restraint and grace in the female role. Read the following details first.

The No walk – suriashi

One of the key principles of the No actor is the sense of being connected at all times to the ground, being 'earthed'. Before performances, No apprentices are responsible for cleaning and polishing the stage – a sacred site – and only the initiated may walk upon it. Thus, the simple act of walking on the stage has weighty significance, and it follows that there are strict rules (conventions) about how to walk. 'The No dancer is weighted in his hips, which remain motionless, as does his torso. The immobile trunk, alive and alert, acts as the energy nexus from which arm and leg movements generate. From skull to tailbone, the straight spine is suspended, so to speak, between heaven and earth. The chin is tucked in and pulled back, giving an extra lift to the back of the skull and an elegance to the unbroken line of the torso' (Bethe and Brazell 25). Stamping when turning, and for effect, is also important. Large ceramic jars are placed at intervals underneath the No stage so that the actor can make stamping movements resonate for extra effect.

'To achieve the gliding walk, the dancer slides one foot along the floor keeping the entire sole in contact with the boards. When he has completed this forward motion, he raises, then lowers the front part of the foot, leaving the heel on the floor to serve as fulcrum. The toes never bend as they rise and fall; the foot always works as a flat unit. Even when stepping forward and shifting the weight from one foot to another, the heels remain on or very close to the floor' (Bethe and Brazell 26).

Restraint

While all roles walk in the suriashi style, this exploration deals with the performance of the female roles only. Giving advice on how to perform female roles, Zeami writes:

> What is felt in the heart is Ten. What appears in movement Seven. When you feel ten in your heart, express seven in your movements . . . in terms of general stage deportment, no matter how slight a bodily action, if the motion is more restrained than the emotion behind it, the emotion will become the Substance and the movements of the body its Function, thus moving the audience. (Zeami 75)

Zeami continues,

> In terms of dance, 'the eyes look ahead and the spirit looks behind.' This expression means that the actor looks in front of him with his physical eyes, but his inner concentration must be directed to the appearance of his movements from behind. This is a crucial element in the creation of what I have referred to as the Movement beyond Consciousness. The appearance of the actor, seen from the spectator in the seating area, produces a different image than the actor can have of himself. What the spectator sees is the outer image of the actor. What an actor himself sees, on the other hand, forms his own internal image of himself. He must make still another effort in order to grasp his own internalized outer image a step possible only through assiduous training. Once he obtains this, the actor and the spectator can share the same image. Only then can it actually be said that an actor has truly grasped the nature of his appearance. For an actor to grasp his true appearance implies that he has under his control the space to the left and to the right of him, and to the front and to the rear of him. In many cases, however, an average actor looks only to the front and to the side and so never sees what he actually looks like from behind. If the actor cannot somehow come to a sense of how he looks from behind, he will not be able to become conscious of any possible vulgarities in his performance. Therefore, an actor must look at himself

using his internalized outer image, come to share the same view as the audience, examine his appearance with his spiritual eyes and so maintain a graceful appearance with his entire body. (Zeami 81)

Grace – Yugen

Zeami claims that the aesthetic quality of grace is considered the highest ideal of perfection (Zeami 92). The word *yugen* means literally 'deep and remote, secluded, dim, quiet, tranquil, serene, of the nether world' and black, dark, mysterious. 'When it comes to playing the role of a woman . . . an actor must concentrate his attention on producing an inner intensity and abandon any detailed stress on his physical movements' (Zeami 141).

Choose either the walk – suriashi; or the concept of restraint or grace and watch a clip from one of the following performances online:

Hagoromo's final dance in Hagoromo (Hagoromo).

Yamamba's kuse dance in Yamamba (Bethe and Brazell 1999).

Atsumori's final dance in Atsumori (Atsumori's Final Dance Before Leaving the Stage).

Watch closely and analyse the aspect you have chosen – either walk or restraint and grace. It may help to take screenshots of particular moments and then draw on the image with labels or arrows to show how the movement or action is made.

Choose a favourite female character from a familiar story, TV show, film or play and a specific moment of emotion from which to develop a movement piece of less than 90 seconds. Explore how to interpret this character physically by applying, adapting or modifying either the walk or restraint and grace as they are used in No theatre. Share and give feedback. What aesthetic changes need to be made to turn the figure into a No role?

In conclusion, whole-class reckoning

Is feminine physicality fixed? Is feminine physicality the same in different parts of the world/history? Do the shape and movement of the body affect the feelings and inner workings of the mind? How can the stage mirror synthesis and harmony of an idea as well as synthesis of gender?

Resources, No theatre

"Atsumori's Final Dance Before Leaving the Stage." February 2012. *YouTube.* January 2020. <https://youtu.be/Yan0TpfOQMM>.

Bethe, Monica and Karen Brazell. "Dance in the No Theater." *Cornell East Asia Series* 1.29 (1982).

—. "Subtitled Video of Noh Theatre Performance of Yamamba 1999." 2006. *Cornell University Library.* January 2020. <https://hdl.handle.net/1813/3339>.

Bogart, Anne and Tina Landau. *The Viewpoints Book.* New York: Theatre Communications Group, 2006.

Riley, Jo. *Chinese Theatre and the Actor in Performance.* Cambridge: Cambridge University Press, 1997.

Zeami. *On the Art of the No Drama, the Major Treatises of Zeami transl. J Thomas Rimer and Yamazaki Makazu.* Princeton, NJ: Princeton University Press, 1984.

"Hagoromo." 2018. *Asian Traditional Theatre and Dance.* February 2020. <https://disco.teak.fi/asia/hagoromo/>.

Kabuki

The usual translation of the words ka-bu-ki simply means song-dance-theatre, although it is possible that similar sounding, but different characters had the meaning 'to incline, to tilt to one side' meaning 'unusual' and 'unconventional'. This points to the essence of a Kabuki show – it is high fashion, 'extravagant, spectacular and faddish, even avant-garde' (Gunji 17). It arose in the early 1600s from earlier dance entertainments and is markedly different from earlier styles of Japanese theatre such as No, in part because the performers are not masked. The Kabuki stage has multiple levels, platforms, steps and catwalk-like gangways through the audience to the stage (hanamichi). The Kabuki also introduced extensive traps, lifts and the revolving stage as well as multiple backdrops and sudden-reveal curtains. The plays are either historical, focusing on warriors and nobles, or contemporary, focusing on sensational murder, adultery and love-suicides. Many of these stories were originally written for the puppet theatre, Bunraku. Thus, in some plays, there is a narrator sitting at the side of the stage and musicians are also present onstage. It is likely that Kabuki was performed to teach good manners and good conduct, whether how to 'visit a brothel, or how a warrior's wife should crush insolence or defend her young mistress from villainy, or the proper way of exacting revenge' (Dunn and Torigo 23)

Performers

The cast is all male. Young boys are trained by older actors in private schools. The acting is stylized, non-naturalistic, physically and vocally demanding and requires mastery of movement, including martial arts, and vocal recitation. There are conventionalized exits and entrances called roppo and still images at the climax of emotion called mie. The actors execute complicated and sudden costume transformations on stage and black-clothed stagehands called kurogo help them do this, as well as passing props and adjusting the fall of the costume when the actor sits or kneels. Performers of traditional-style Kabuki use a type of make-up called kumadori which uses bold lines of red and/or blue on white that are influenced by facial expressions on Buddhist statues and No theatre masks. Red lines might indicate virtue or strength and blue is used for evil. The costumes and make-up are spectacularly exaggerated in colour, form and line, and actors wear elaborate wigs because even hair conveys 'religious significance, status significance, married status and is a means of expressing beauty' (Dunn and Torigo 49).

Audience

The audience comprises all members of society and because performances might continue from dawn to dusk, the audience might walk in and out throughout the day. The auditorium can be noisy, with shouts of approval from the audience to the stage at moments of great skill; chatting with one another, and eating and drinking throughout is common. Most of the plays are well known to the audiences, so they look forward to the best bits and chat through the less interesting parts. Moreover, many Kabuki plays were written to celebrate a specific actor's skills, and the audience generally know not only which actor's specific skills to applaud, but also each actor's training history and acting heritage. They are a rowdy, but expert, audience.

Men playing women - the onnagata

The actor playing a female role is known as an onna-gata (literally female-in-form; it's the same term for kata or pattern above). Unlike the No theatre, Kabuki actors tend to specialize in one role category. Yoshizawa Ayame (1673–1729), a famed player of women's roles, wrote a collection of notes and advice by Kabuki actors, and a list of these actors and the parts they played, translated as The Actor's Analects. He claims only men can know how to perform the onnagata role:

> If an actress were to appear on the stage, she could not express the ideal feminine beauty, for she would rely only on the exploitation of her physical characteristics, and therefore not express the synthetic ideal. The ideal woman can only be expressed by an actor. (Ernst 195)

Ayame repeatedly suggests that the best onnagata live as females offstage, although they may be married and have children. He believed that living as a woman would feed the onstage presentation with a certain 'mysterious mood' (Leiter, Frozen Moments 15). However, the question of 'becoming' or simply 'representing' another gender is not clear-cut, despite Ayame. There are always moments in Kabuki where the onnagata deliberately displays masculine qualities before suddenly checking herself and shifting to more feminine movements (Leiter, From Gay to Gei 509). The audience recognizes these moments and enjoys them. It is like a moment of belief/disbelief, where the audience sees both real and not-real simultaneously. Is this the source of delight in watching the onnagata? In many ways, it could be said that gender is like a repeated stylization of the body – a set of repeated acts that become engrained. The audience is fully aware of the male actor behind the representation of the female role. Generally, the onnagata part is somewhat sedate. Sometimes, however, the onnagata has a solo dance piece where she can express her deepest feelings choreographically. These are emotional highlights for onnagata and may include chastising someone for an injustice, saying farewell to a beloved, or weeping for a dead child (Leiter, From Gay to Gei 503). Table 5.1 shows various instructions from Ayame's Manual on how to be a perfect onnagata.

Table 5.1 Ayame's instructions on how to perform onnagata (Dunn and Torigo)

'In onnagata playing, her outward appearance should be coquettish, but her heart chaste. And to make a samurai's wife unfeminine just because she is a samurai's wife is bad acting. When one is playing the role of a strong-minded woman, one must see that her heart has some softness' (Dunn and Torigo 51).	'The onnagata role has its basis in charm, and even one who has innate beauty, if he seeks to make a fine show in a fighting scene, will lose the femininity of his performance. Or again, if he tries deliberately to make his interpretation elegant, it will not be pleasing. For these reasons, if he does not live his normal life as if he was a woman, it will not be possible for him to be called a skilful onnagata. The more an actor is persuaded that it is the time when he appears on stage that is the most important in his career as an onnagata, the more masculine he will be. It is better for him to consider his everyday life as the most important' (Dunn and Torigo 53).
'The onnagata should continue to have the feelings of an onnagata even when in the dressing room. When taking refreshment, too, he should turn away so that people cannot see him' (Dunn and Torigo 61).	'First of all, the male character must always be in the forefront, the female behind. There is an imaginary line on the stage behind which the onnagata must stay. This is because of feudalistic attitudes . . . the woman must do everything in a reserved manner, underplaying, never exerting her full external energies' (Leiter, Frozen Moments 14).

Table 5.1 Continued

'In the case of the wife of an elder counsellor threatening an enemy, the actor has in mind that she is the wife of a samurai and so always has her place her hand on her sword in a haughty fashion. To play her as too bold in the handling of a sword, when, for all that she is a samurai's wife, she does not normally wear such a weapon, is bad acting. The best way to portray her is that she should not be afraid of her sword' (Dunn and Torigo 50).	'It goes without saying that an onnagata performance should hold the audience through the heart. When standing, the actor should have his feet turned inwards. The waist should be slender and the opening of skirts just right ... Notes: onnagata used a pigeon-toed (the text says crocodile) stance ... the kimono opens into an inverted V over the feet, affording a glimpse of the under kimono. It is important that this opening should be neither too small nor too large' (Dunn and Torigo 159).
'Among the things that I heard Ayame say to Jujiro was this "My friend, I congratulate you upon the popularity that you are enjoying from your audiences, but you must give up any deliberate attempt to make them laugh ... Trying to make audiences laugh is no part of womanly feeling"' (Dunn and Torigo 54).	'To be alongside a tachiyaku playing the lover's part, and chew away at one's food without charm and then go straight out on the stage and play a love scene with the same man, will lead to failure on both sides' (Dunn and Torigo 61).
Some renowned onnagata actors were: Asao Jijiro (died 1635) Hashimoto Kinsaku (dates unknown c.1655) Ichimura Tamagashiwa (no dates) Iwai Heijiro (last decade of the 17th century) Kirinami Senju (flourished 1710) Kokan Taroji (died 1713) Mizuki Tatsumosuke (1673–1745) Namie Kokan (born 1659) Okada Samanosuke (flourished 1680–1700) Sodeshima Genji (flourished 1699) Tamiya Shirogoro (1685–1745) Yoshizawa Ayame (1673–1729) (Dunn and Torigo 174–194).	'Yamashita was asked about the acting of onnagata parts and replied: "There are three very important rules for the onnagata. His acting towards a man with whom the character he is playing is in love should be very reserved and he should be reticent about it. In his acting, when it seems that the man has fallen in love, first, it is better that the onnagata should be unrestrainedly harsh. Over and above these two rules, it is extremely important that no matter how he is urged by the writer of the play, he should refuse to act in it if it has some situation that involves a departure from womanly modesty"' (Dunn and Torigo 121)
'The onnagata wear layers of costume, headdress, wig and wooden clogs. The onnagata occasionally alter their way of walking by dragging the inside edges of their clogs in a sweeping figure (hachimonji). This movement requires that they slightly open the legs which are otherwise always pressed together shifting her role towards the seductive' (Leiter, From Gay to Gei 499).	A key aspect of Kabuki is 'Puppet gesture ... a specific choreography in which a human performer moves as if he or she were a bunraku puppet. Puppet-gesture tends to be used by women characters in a short sequence usually at the climax of a piece ... when beginning the sequence, the actor-dancer suddenly becomes a puppet, falling into complete silence, erasing facial expression and muting footsteps ... the lines of the character ... are spoken by a narrator ... the actor's body from head to toe is manipulated by other actors playing the roles of the puppeteers and footsteps are provided by one of the puppeteers stamping the floor' (Isaka 104).

Excavation One – onnagata female-in-form

Choose one of the following onnagata dance sequences from the plays to watch online:

Musume Dojoji or Dojoji Temple (Kabuki at 9.00; Bando from 4.33).
Fuji Musume or Wisteria Maiden (Wisteria Maiden).
Narukami or Thunder God (Ichikawa).
Sagi Musume or The Heron Maiden (Sagi Musume; Heron Maiden).
Kinkakuji or The Golden Pavilion (kinkakuji).
Read a synopsis first, then watch the video sequence.

Choose either: pose, fan or props and select a 30-second clip from the video to study more closely. Use slow-motion replay or make screenshots of each movement in order to break the sequence down. Have a go at replicating the sequence. You can film yourself and match each section to the screengrabs you made. Ask a friend to watch and give feedback.

Survey the terrain

What are the elements of Kabuki female-in-form; how are they put together and how do they work together in one body?

Musume Dojoji or Dojoji Temple

A young girl has fallen in love with a priest who is, naturally, forbidden to return her love. The young girl's love turns to hate, and she transforms into a fire-breathing serpent. In fear, the priest hides inside a giant temple bell. The girl-serpent wraps herself around the bell and sets it alight so that the priest is burnt to death and the bell melts away. The dance begins at the temple, with the bell in place, centre stage. There are cherry blossoms all around, and the girl performs a sedate dance from the No theatre to honour the temple bell. The actor makes a fast change in costume on stage (hikinuki) from red to pale blue and portrays a woman in love whose love is unrequited. There are several more transitions to different costumes and moods of love before she arrives at a lilac costume with a hand towel between her teeth as a sign of distress, disappointment and other feelings of jealousy. From here, she changes into a yellow costume, beating a hand drum and dances like the spirit fox. Another costume switch turns the costume white, and she holds two drums as her face changes expression. She releases the outer red garment and reveals the scaly costume underneath before climbing onto the bell and venting her anger. Sometimes, the middle scenes are omitted from the performance.

Fuji Musume or Wisteria Maiden

The play is set in Otsu, outside the ancient capital of Kyoto, where tourists like to come and buy paintings of the surrounding countryside. A gentleman passer-by spies a painting of a wisteria flower maiden. The maiden in the painting immediately falls in love with him and comes to life, holding a branch of the wisteria and wearing a black lacquered hat. She dances to show unrequited love; drinks sake after depicting a lover's tiff; and writes a love letter with emotions of hopelessness, before returning to the painting. The piece also involves a moment of hikinuki fast costume change.

Narukami or Thunder God

Narukami is a priest who has caused the empire great drought because in a drunken rage he locked the dragon king (god of rain) behind a waterfall. Princess Taema is sent to save the day which she does in a dance lifting her skirts to entice the priest. As they are alone, Taema pretends to faint, and Narukami catches her, accidentally touching her breast. He is infatuated with her, so she makes him increasingly drunk so that she can cut the rope and free the dragon.

Sagi Musume or the Heron Maiden

A young girl has died with a bitter heart and turned into the spirit of a heron. The play starts in mid-winter. She performs a dance with several sections including hikinuki costume changes: the first section of the dance is the young maiden in love wearing a red kimono to show her joy in love. This is followed by a blue costume and a cheeky folk song suggesting it is harder to love someone than scoop salt from the sea, then a lively parasol dance, and, finally, her punishment in hell as her bird-self returns, reincarnated, with blood on her shoulder and a willow leaf in her hand.

Kinkakuji or the Golden Pavilion

This Kabuki play was originally a puppet drama from the Bunraku theatre. The evil Daizhen is sitting playing Go and challenges young Tokichi. When Tokichi wins, Daizhen sets him three impossible tasks, which Tokichi also achieves. Daizhen demands Princess Yuki should paint a dragon on the ceiling of the Golden Pavilion, but she gives him reasons not to do so, one of which is that she loves her husband. In a rage, Daizhen threatens to kill her husband, but Yuki grabs a sword and attacks him. For this, she is tied to a cherry tree and her husband is condemned to death. As Yuki's husband is led past her, the cherry blossoms fall to the earth. She uses her foot to draw a picture of mice in the blossoms, and these mice come to life and gnaw at her ropes to free her. Tokichi takes up the sword and kills Daizhen.

Kabuki loves spectacle, and the Kabuki stage is packed with secret traps, revolves, reveals and scenic transformations. According to Samuel Leiter, these included

Excavation Two – Hikinuki onstage transformations

In three of the plays mentioned above – Dojoji Temple Maiden, Wisteria Maiden and Heron Maiden – the actor portrays a different mood and emotion in the dance by making a fast costume change on stage. Choose one of these and watch the moment of costume change very carefully. A kurogo or stage assistant is unobtrusively present to help. The kurogo is said to be as skilful a performer as the dancer. Look at the brief demonstration of how this can be done in the video of Wisteria Maiden. Using contemporary stage costume, can you and a partner recreate a dramatic moment of costume change onstage? First, establish the scene and character for at least 30 seconds before the costume change; then continue the new outward appearance of the character for at least 30 seconds after the transformation.

Set the compass

The outer form, costume, shapes, props and movement of the onnagata reveal inner emotions which change when the hikinuki transformation onstage is completed.

The outer form, shapes and movement of the onnagata change how the actor feels on the inside.

The outer form, shapes and movement of the onnagata are received by the audience as representations of the female role regardless of the gender of the actor portraying them.

Legless ghosts . . . suspended in mid-air, (who) rose from water, or slid on their bellies through lanterns; bodies continued moving after being cut in half; people metamorphosed into skeletons; giant cats, frogs, and boa constrictors breathed fire; realistic rain fell in torrents; swords pierced characters' necks; sets changed in the twinkling of an eye; living heads rolled around in flaming wheels; buildings collapsed. (Leiter, Frozen Moments 94)

One key technique of spectacle is the 'Kabuki drop', doncho, which is created by a pale blue/green curtain called asagimaku. The curtain is very light, undecorated and has no folds. Often, there will be a short scene or prologue in front of this curtain, and the percussion rhythm increases in pace before a sudden silence and the curtain falls to the floor to reveal a spectacularly colourful or different scene behind. The technique is called furiotoshi, which means 'shake off' describing the movement of the curtain as it shivers to the floor. The drop curtain is not used at a moment of emotional intensity or climax, but more likely, sometime after the main climax has been reached – it is not a dramatic reveal, despite it's being used globally now to reveal the latest model at automobile exhibitions.

Other curtain techniques are the main draw curtain, hikimaku, in persimmon, green and black stripes. The curtain does not mark the beginning and the end of the performance, but rather moments of pause and reflection – at the end of the play Kanjincho, the hikimaku closes the stage area so that Benkei, the hero, can make a spectacular exit along the hanamachi bridge. The hikimaku curtain is drawn to and from stage left by an invisible curtain puller.

Keshimaku is a disappearing curtain, which allows actors, especially those who have been executed or killed, to exit without being seen, when a red cloth is used to indicate they are dead. There is also a 'mist' curtain or kasumimaku that hides musicians or performers temporarily not involved in the main scene. This curtain is usually blue and white with images of clouds on it.

Another curtain technique is the kuromaku or black curtain used as backdrop in the play, The Forest of Suzu (Suzugamori) to indicate the night-time.

The drop curtain technique can be seen in the play:

Yoshitsune Sembon Zakura – Yoshitsune and the Thousand Cherry Trees (Authentic Kabuki with Commentary 1:19:00–1:22:00)

Excavation Three – the Kabuki drop or doncho

Take a familiar story from a folk tale and identify a moment in the plot where the Kabuki drop might be especially effective. Consider your intentions for this moment – to shock, to surprise, to delight . . . What must happen before and after the Kabuki drop to ensure its full effect?

Practically explore how to execute the Kabuki drop for your chosen moment. Can you find a low-tech solution?

Explore the lighting situation for your Kabuki drop. Will you use projections or coloured light on your reveal curtain? Investigate how to use a 'scrim' where the position of the light source affects transparency. Explore music and/or sound effect in combination with the Kabuki drop moment.

Document your findings in a series of photographs/illustrations with annotations to comment on effectiveness, problems, solutions.

In conclusion, whole-class reckoning

Consider the role of technology in creating and transforming identities on stage.

Resources, Kabuki

"Atsumori's Final Dance Before Leaving the Stage." February 2012. *YouTube*. January 2020. <https://youtu.be/Yan0TpfOQMM>.

"Authentic Kabuki with Commentary." 29 June 2018. *YouTube*. April 2020. <https://youtu.be/senRJ0KJ7rE>.

Bando, Tamasaburo. "Musume Dojoji." 4 August 2018. *YouTube*. April 2020. <https://youtu.be/G6NCR2AJE0I>.

Dunn, Charles and Bunzo Torigo. *The Actors' Analects, Edited Translated and with an Introduction.* Ed. Charles J. Dunn and Bunzo Torigoe. Columbia: Columbia University Press, 1969.

Ernst, Earle. *The Kabuki Theatre*. Honolulu: University of Hawaii Press, 1974.

Gunji, Masakatsu. *The Kabuki Guide*. Tokyo: Kodansha International, 1987.

"Heron Maiden." 13 November 2011. *YouTube*. April 2020. <https://youtu.be/6q_sbK2sfPM>.

"kinkakuji." n.d. *Kabuki Play Guide*. April 2020. http://enmokudb.kabuki.ne.jp/repertoire_en/the-golden-pavilion%ef%bc%88kinkakuji%ef%bc%89

Leiter, Samuel J. "From Gay to Gei." *Comparative Drama* (1999–2000): 495–514.

—. *Frozen Moments*. New York: Cornell University Press, 2002.

"Sagi Musume." 4 January 2014. *YouTube*. April 2020. <https://youtu.be/d7xYC1maiU4>.

"Wisteria Maiden." 8 November 2006. *YouTube*. April 2020. <https://youtu.be/sPgtX-ljHi4>.

"Wisteria Maiden." 4 April 2007. *YouTube*. April 2020. <https://youtu.be/72IjyxGU8sk>.

Takarazuka – female actors playing men

Takarazuka is a musical revue entertainment named after a hot spring spa town at the end of the Hankyu Railway Line from Osaka. In 1914, the president of the Hanyku Railway, Ichizo Kobayashi, initiated the entertainment as a tourist attraction to encourage city dwellers out into the spa region to relax and enjoy entertainment. The Takarazuka Revue Company started with 18 young girls and now has 5 huge companies of 400 – the performers are all girls. The Takarazuka performances are mostly exotic, flamboyant, melodramatic and musical adaptations of Western stories, novels and films such as Cinderella, Wuthering Heights, The Count of Monte Cristo, Guys and Dolls, Casablanca or Oceans 11. The plots mostly involve triangular love affairs, unrequited love, danger and tragedy, or are spectacular revues without plot. The Takarazuka is a fantasy world; a melodrama full of daring and adventure, love, passion and tortured romance (Robertson 226).

Performers

Young female actors train in singing, dancing, acting and traditional Japanese dance at the Takarazuka Music School for two years. Students are assigned a role category, either female roles – musemeyaku, or male roles – otokoyaku. Museme means daughter; otoko means man. Although the female actor provided a vehicle to represent or enact the idea of an ideal man, the otokoyaku was not considered to be male or to represent the idea of male for others to imitate in life. In Kabuki, the term kata in onnagata means 'model' or 'archetype' of female; in Takarazuka the 'yaku' word suggests task, job or duty to be executed as a solider might execute the general's commands. 'The female who plays a man is but performing a duty' (Robertson 59). The performer must over-exaggerate the look of a male by showing excessive markers of masculinity – the more stereotyped the better. It is a theatricalization of the stereotypical (and fictional) male (Robertson 259).

The style of Takarazuka is deliberately over-exaggerated and melodramatic and verges on Camp, explored in Chapter 4. 'The essence of Camp is love of the unnatural: of artifice and exaggeration' (Sontag 275). It is 'a sensibility that . . . converts the serious into the frivolous . . . a certain mode of aestheticism. It is *one* way of seeing the world as an aesthetic phenomenon' (Sontag 227). This is a deliberate choice that makes style more important than content (plot) or character development, or certainly 'message'. In this sense, the performances can be seen as 'pure artifice' (Sontag 281), and audiences revel in this consciously artificially upheld view of the world. In the same way that Kabuki has been termed sensationalist and Hollywood-style (Leims), so Takarazuka has been accused of being 'nylon Kabuki' (Robertson 226) because similar aesthetic principles of exaggeration, sensationalism and synthetic entertainment apply.

Audience

The audience is composed almost entirely of women, and there is a vast fan club of women of all ages. In the past, a Japanese woman was only considered female if married and a mother. Unmarried females were known as shojo, which means literally 'not quite female'. Within the shojo group of unmarried girls are gyaru (sounds like 'gal'), used for older females, and ojin gyaru (older-man gal) that refers to girls who sing karaoke and drink in bars. Another term for the Takarazuka spectator is moga, which means modern girl. These are the new working women – females far from the ideals of traditional Good Wife and Wise Mother (Robertson 265).

Excavation One – stereotyping the male role

Browse the official Takarazuka website (Revue) for some background information, videos and images. Other videos are available online and on DVD. Female actors crossdressing as males in the Takarazuka involves framing: specific elements that are thought to represent masculinity are selected and put together in deliberate ways. However, the audience is always aware that the performer is female, and, indeed, there are some markers of femininity in the composition of the male role. This makes their performance ambiguous, as belonging to both masculine and feminine roles.

What are the key signifiers of the otokoyaku representation of the male? Using 2 of Kowzan's 13 signs of theatre as in Table 5.2, choose one character from the website's gallery to analyse an otokoyaku character from a performance.

Table 5.2 Organizer to map otokoyaku outward signs of appearance

	Element	Evidence	What does it mean in the performance?
Actor's external appearance	1. make-up		
	2. hair		
	3. costume		
Appearance of the stage	4. props		

In groups of three to four, take 90 seconds to write down as many favourite movies you can think of. Take a moment to consider all the titles, then in another 90 seconds choose ONE movie together.

Now refine the cast of your chosen movie to three to four key roles and, as a group, start to discuss the key features of each, using the role-on-the-wall technique.

Choose ONE character each to design individually. Some of the characteristics you have noted as a group in the role-on-the-wall should be represented in costume and props. These must now be over-exaggerated by you as the designer. If a prince's cloak is an essential aspect then fur, colour, length can be emphasized – think about size, proportion, colour intensity, texture. Your design must not be comical; it must be stylish, cool; and it can be Camp.

Some of the characteristics you have noted in the Role-on-the-Wall exercise may be inner, psychological feelings or experiences of the character. Can your design include any of these internal aspects on the outside – in costume? They should be immediately recognizable – there is nothing subtle about Takarazuka.

If you haven't already done so, now consider the specific location and time period of your piece. How can these be reflected in your costume design?

Survey the terrain

Collate the individual sketches and ideas from the group into a 'gallery' for your own website advertising this play.

Excavation Two – intention and action

Intention: in the same groups, discuss your designs and ideas and pull them together into a cohesive design – location and period; colour palette, line. As a group, create a logline for advertising your show online. A logline includes a description of the protagonist in one word, and the protagonist's goal is briefly outlined. The antagonist is described in one action word, followed by an outline of the stakes or conflict and finishing with a teaser ending.

For example: successful Scottish whiskey distiller must marry before his father dies to ensure inheritance while jealous stepmother poisons city water to stop him. Bride-to-be works at the city waterworks and loves a bagpipe playing, impoverished engineer from the oil rigs. How long can the city survive? Will love overcome the tartan clan clash?

Add the logline as title to your 'gallery'.

Action

You have designed a role for your character from the outside in. In pairs, you must find a way to realize the costume in practice. Choose pieces of costume, adding padding, or layering, as necessary to realize your design in practice. The costume may restrict, shape, define or liberate movements in the role. Bearing this in mind, now that the costume is complete, experiment with:

Stance – a simple standing posture that characterizes the role immediately for the audience.

Walk – how does the character walk?

A typical gesture made by the character.

A typical phrase or sentence spoken by the character.

A piece of music or sound effect that conjures the essence of your character that might play in the background when your character appears.

Remember, the goal of the creation of character is to appeal to a young and stylish audience. The character should not become a cartoon figure of fun but an ultra-stylish, cool figure to admire. Take photos to add to the 'gallery'.

Individual compass

Choose one of these topics to create a podcast of maximum 2 minutes to discuss your thoughts on:

Stereotype.

The aesthetic of Camp.

Inner/outer representations of a role.

In conclusion, whole-class reckoning

Who has authority to determine the conventions of performing a particular gender? Must the performance of gender be 'believable' in theatre, or is it merely representation? Who has authority to grant 'believability' in theatre performance? How might this apply to real life?

Resources, Takarazuka

Leims, Thomas. "Kabuki goes to Hollywood. Reforms and 'Revues' in the 1980s." *The Dramatic Touch of Difference: Theatre, Own and Foreign*. Ed. Erika Fischer-Lichte, Josephine Riley and Michael Gissenwehrer. Tübingen Gunter Narr, 1990. 107–119

Revue, Takarazuka. "Takarazuka Revue." 2020. *Takarazuka Revue.* April 2020. <https://kageki.hankyu.co.jp/english/index.html>.

Robertson, Jennifer. *Takarazuka, Sexual Politics and Popular Culture in Modern Japan.* Berkeley: University of California Press, 1998.

Sontag, Susan. *'Notes on Camp' in Against Interpretation.* New York: Farrar, Straus and Giroux, 1961.

Yueju – women playing men playing women

The Chinese traditional theatre has been the domain of male actors after various imperial bans on female performers since 1671 by the Kangxi emperor and finally after the ultimate ban on women performers in 1774. Women did perform unofficially in tea houses and brothels, and it was this association that prevented female actors from being included in professional theatre performances as they were considered lewd and bawdy. There were no mixed-gender acting troupes. During the Qing dynasty (1644–1911) and Republican period (1912–1949), the theatre scene was dominated by male performers and, particularly, the fame and prominence of four great female impersonators, see below. Despite their fame, and considerably larger wages than the rest of the company, however, the actor specializing in female roles 'was not permitted to sit on the dressing boxes backstage or walk in front of actors playing male roles when the troupe hiked to the next site' (Jin 231). The most famous male actors of female roles in Jingju are: Mei Lanfang, Cheng Yanqiu, Shang Xiaoyun and Xun Huisheng.

The situation changed dramatically with the opening of the trade ports Shanghai and Ningbo, the growth of Foreign (Western) Concessions and a flow of immigrants from the countryside to urban centres seeking a livelihood after the 1930 great depression in the silk trade. The foreign settlements, 'physically and conceptually marked as separate, offered some of the earliest venues for female actors, despite attempts by Chinese authorities to regulate the performances' (Goodman and Larson 44). The May 4th New Culture Movement introduced in the 1920s during the Republican Era also promoted equality in the workplace, including the condemnation of both arranged marriages and the practice of concubinage. Similarly, Chinese scholars who travelled to Japan returned to China with new ideas about naturalist, spoken drama as practiced in the West, breaking the hold of traditional theatre forms. Finally, the outbreak of the war of resistance against Japan in 1937 aided the rise of women into the public arena, since restrictions on female performers were lifted by the Japanese occupiers. In fact, the Japanese authorities were keen to support the idea of women's liberation, since it was thought to promote Japan's modernist outlook.

Under these conditions, a new form of theatre developed, based on folk melodies and instrumentation, performed entirely by all-female troupes. It was named Yueju after the geographical area of its birth around Shanghai. It is very different from the Yueju theatre from Guangdong/Canton which uses different Chinese characters in its name, although it sounds similar. A record of Shanghai theatre performances on one night in 1938 shows that there were 2 naturalistic plays, 3 performances of the local Shanghai opera, 1 of the elite-style Kunqu, 12 performances of Jingju and 12 of Yueju (Jin 219) confirming the immense popularity of Yueju. As popular media such as radio and cinema grew, the popularity of the actors playing Yueju also increased. Female actors performed regularly on radio from 1939, and profited from the new media by advertising soap, tonics and cosmetics and appearing in fan magazines and playbills, alongside printed lyrics of the arias and personal details of their lives.

As a regional style of traditional Chinese theatre, Yueju includes song, recitation, acting and martial arts just like Jingju, but its dialect is local to the Zhejiang area and its melodies and instrumentation are also of the region. It started in Eastern Zhejiang Province in an area known in earlier times as Yue in the early 1900s as itinerant players performed at temple fairs, gambling dens, tea houses and village markets for a small fee. The troupes were made up of all-male, then all-child actors and later all-female actors. The stages they performed on were makeshift, temporary structures, open on all sides. Much of the Yue area is intersected by rivers and canals, and often the temples built at the harbour edge or canal side included stages where spectators could view the performance from the water in boats. On one occasion, the owner of a local cloth shop sent five sedan chairs to bring a group of young performers to perform at his mother's birthday celebration. 'The troupe travelled or rather paraded, about twenty five miles in sedan chairs, stopping to perform at several places and causing a sensation on the way' (Jin 256).

By the 1920s, Yueju had moved into urban cities like Shanghai, and the child troupes gradually developed into all-girl troupes which were highly popular. In Shanghai, Yueju was performed in fixed theatre buildings with a proscenium arch as well as tea house theatres. At the same time, Yueju actors improved its repertoire and musical sophistication from rural folk style to more elevated, sophisticated use of music and language (Jin 26). Yueju schools were established around the entire Zhejiang area, and young peasant girls strove to become Yueju actors as a means of escaping rural poverty. The Yueju repertoire developed in the late 1930s and 1940s from patriotic and modernist reform plays, family morality plays and erotic plays to the romantic love plays for which Yueju is now mostly known. There is an extreme contrast between Jingju and Yueju. Yueju is considered soft and flexible following the Yin principle, while Jingju is considered masculine and tough like the principle of Yang. The costumes and movements in Yueju are not conventionalized like Jingju, and the romantic plots may be set in the past or present with historical or contemporary costumes. A chorus sometimes sings backstage to set the scene and comment on the action.

The actors

Historically, actors in China belonged to the lowest social class, the three 'zi': 'actors' (xizi), soldiers (liangzi) and prostitutes (biaozi). Yuan Xuefen, female actor of female roles, reports on her childhood:

> The year I was 11 years old (1933) I started at the Four Seasons Theatre School. When studying and travelling to perform in Shaoxing, Zhuji, Hangzhou, Ningbo, Shanghai and various other places, for eight years of my life I felt keenly that the theatre troupe was the epitome of the old society, and society was at its lowest level, and wherever I went I could see that the weak were at the mercy of the strong. Subjected at home and abroad to attack from both sides, very few of my fellow sister actors were able to escape being broken. You could count on your fingers the few girls who managed to struggle through the suffering before facing defeat and giving up entirely. (Yuan 3)

At 14, Yuan Xuefen was pushed onto centre stage although she was still learning the part. However, there were no scripts and the plays relied on instant improvisation which made it especially difficult for this young girl to succeed. Yuan calls this training 'a battlefield' (Yuan 4). Later, even in Shanghai, the female actors were entirely controlled by male theatre managers. Yuan states, 'The bosses . . . had ideas that were very different from mine. They would consider nothing but their profit' (Jin 275). Yuan Xuefen specialized in female roles, and although she does not really belong in this chapter, she is important to mention here since she was selected by Zhou Enlai, Vice Chairman of the Communist Party, to participate in the first session of the Chinese People's Political Conference Committee in 1946 alongside two of the great male actors of female roles: Mei Lanfang and Cheng Yanqiu. Later, on 1 October 1949, when Chairman Mao proclaimed the founding of the People's Republic of China, Yuan Xuefen was the guest of Zhou Enlai and stood at the top of Tiananmen Gate (see Figure 5.5). Her attempts to reform Yueju, promoting women's rights, earned her a prominent position in Chinese politics (Yuan 121–125).

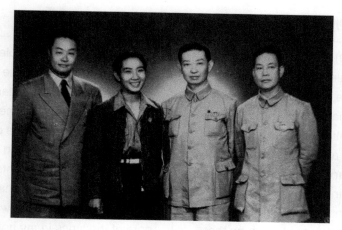

Figure 5.5 From left: Cheng Yanqiu, Yuan Xuefen, Mei Lanfang and Zhou Xinfang represent actors at the Political Conference Committee (Yuan 67).

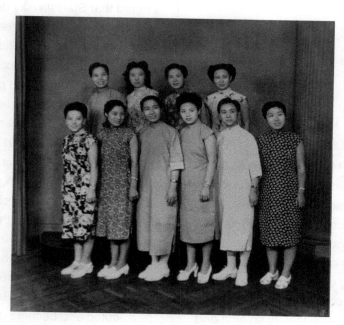

Figure 5.6 The Ten Sisters actor collaborative (Yuan 61).

In the 1930s, the 'four great male actors of female roles' of Jingju were matched by the 'three flowers and one grace' of Yueju (*hua* means flower and *juan* means grace). The most famous female actors of male roles in Yueju are: Shi Yinhua, Tu Xinghua 'more like a man than a man', Zhao Ruihua and Yao Shuijuan. The four outstanding female actors of female roles in Yueju are: Wang Xinghua, Shi Yinhua who sang 'like a bead necklace with countable grains', Zhao Ruihua and Yao Shuijuan. In 1947, several leading actors from different Yueju companies in Shanghai formed the 'Ten Sisters' collaborative (see Figure 5.6).

The Ten Sisters' Collaborative held charity performances to raise money to make radical changes to the way theatre companies were organized. It empowered them to take over the management and administration of their own all-female company and control the repertoire, which had previously been in the hands of somewhat unscrupulous male owners. The actors called each other older sister and younger sister and ran the theatre companies and schools attached to them in a very different style to the hierarchical system run by men. Brief information on the key leading female actors playing male roles is given in Table 5.3.

Table 5.3 Leading Yueju female actors of male roles

Tu Xinghua (1918–1939) was the most famous originator of the female actor of the male role. She specialized in the non-military roles of scholar and civil official. In 1931, she even performed with an entirely male company in Shanghai. Tu was an avid reader and brought new stories and literary works to the stage, which was unusual since most of her acting sisters could not even read. Tu partnered Shi Yinhua, and the pair were known as the Empresses Yin (Silver) and Apricot (Tu). Tu regarded Shi's parents as her own (Tu Xinghua).	Fan Ruijuan (1924–2017) played male roles from the age. The very first role she played was also the one she made most famous- the lover Liang Shanbo in the story of The Butterfly Lovers. As a child, she joined the company of Lan Su E, 'I secretly watched and studied, looking at her expressive movements, and also following her lyrics. When the evening's performance was over, and everyone was asleep, I made a note of the lyrics in my notebook. This method of learning was called 'stealing the play' (Gao 70). Fan Ruijuan also recalls learning about the Stanislavsky System. 'During the 1940s reforms, I heard that Stanislavsky dealt with theatre directing . . .so I started reading. My literacy level was low and theoretical works were difficult for me' but with the help of others, she began to 'study, understand and perform a wide range of characters, especially how to create various characters through our careful observation of people in real life' (Gao 91).
Ma Zhanghua (1927–1942) was known as the 'lightning bolt actor' since her rise to stardom was extremely rapid and brief. Her early death, aged 21, propelled Yueju theatre into the limelight. At the funeral ceremony, 'there were so many people they couldn't all get in, crowds braved deep piercing cold, standing outside the hall, and there were sounds of wailing, choking and sobs. The occasion was very solemn and ceremonial, very seldom seen' (Gao 191). Like nearly all Yueju actors, Ma started out with a traveling performing group. She lived in ruined temples, sleeping on straw, and once was even grabbed from the stage by police (Gao). Ma was a talented tumbler, performing male martial arts roles with ease. When she partnered Yuan Xuefen, they were said to be as 'a necklace of pearls and a girdle of jade' and she was also said to be the first Yueju actor to perform on the radio. She had several adoptive mothers, or wealthy stage patrons, who provided gifts and meals in exchange for reflected fame.	Yin Guifang (1919–2000) was a leading female actor specializing in young male roles. She created a series of roles such as the revolutionary Shi Dakai, the great general of the Taiping Heavenly Kingdom in 1946; the Guangxu Emperor, and Sun Kexian, who fought the invading Qing army (Robertson 96). During the Cultural Revolution, she was persecuted and became paralysed down one side.

(*Continued*)

Table 5.3 Continued

Ma eventually married the son of one of these patrons, and when he demanded that she give up the stage, the theatre owner for whom she worked, realizing his money tree would die out, propagated slander about her character and ruined her reputation, so that she fell ill and died very young.	
Lan Su E (1916–1989) had excellent basic skills and, most particularly, was known for her martial arts and acrobatic skills. Having been trained originally in Jingju techniques, she was renowned for precision and grace.	The Ten Sisters: formed in 1947 at the Atlantic Restaurant in Shanghai, ten of the most prominent Yueju actors created a contract for joint performance to oppose the exploitation of greedy theatre managers. They took unique control of all media and repertoire issues. In Figure 5.6. from left, front row: Xu Tianhong (male role), Fu Quanxiang (female role), Yuan Xuefen,(female role), Zhu Shuizhao (martial arts male and female roles), Fan Ruijuan (male role), Wu Xiaolou (male role), Zhang Guifeng (male role), Xiao Dangui (female role), Xu Yulan (male role) and Yin Guifang (male role).

Audience

In the early 1930s–1940s, most of the Yueju audiences in Shanghai were young schoolgirls, middle-class housewives and the concubines of upper-class men. Later, the large troupes attracted minor intellectuals and scholars (Jin 211). Shanghai was packed with immigrants from all over China seeking work and wealth in the port city. The Yueju actors performed in the local dialect from rural Zhejiang – but its simple and emotional plots meant it had broad appeal. Later, in the 1940s and 1950s, as Yueju reflected theories of equal rights for women and everything modern, the audience was almost entirely composed of schoolgirls, female college students, female professionals and the new middle-class housewives (Jin 212).

The Butterfly Lovers

Mandarin ducks and butterflies are symbols associated with popular romance novels on which the most representative and well-loved plays developed by Yueju female actors, Yuan Xuefen and Fan Ruijuan, were based. The Butterfly Lovers became a poster play in the reform era of the May 4th Movement in the 1920s, promoting women's rights, since it portrays a young girl determined to go to school and become educated and choose her partner in marriage. In its original form, this play was less focused on women's rights and more interested in the erotic play of the main character Zhu, played by a female actor playing a male interacting with Liang, a male scholar played by a female actor dressed as a male. Yuan Xuefen recalls, 'even in a well-developed traditional play such as The Butterfly Lovers, the folklore was riddled with all kinds of feudal superstitions and fatalist trash. . . . There was also a lot of erotic material in the lyric that I felt uncomfortable singing' (Lu and Gao 63). A new scene was added, 'Taking a stand against arranged marriage', and Fan Ruijuan, playing the male lead comments, 'My role as Liang was completely in the hands of the leadership and only under their enlightenment could I break the traditional version of the cute but naughty scoundrel' (Wu 72). Politics and theatre are sometimes inextricable.

Synopsis

The Butterfly Lovers is available online (Liang Shanbo and Zhu Yingtai) and on DVD (directed by Huang Sha in 1954 and Tsui Hark in 1994).

A young girl, Zhu Yingtai, wants to go to school, study the classics and get an education but is prevented from doing this, since she is female. She sets a trap for her father by pretending to be ill from pining to go to college in the city. Her maid asks Yingtai's father to send for a doctor/fortune teller. Yingtai appears in disguise as the male doctor and tells the father that the only way to cure his daughter is to send her to college. Yingtai reveals her disguise as a male and proves that if she were able to fool him into thinking she were a man, then she can use a similar disguise to go to college. Reluctantly, the father agrees. Yingtai and her maid, Yingxin, set out, both dressed in male clothing and, after a while, come to rest at a pavilion. At the same time, a young gentleman scholar, Liang Shanbo, and his servant, are travelling to study at the college, and they, too, come to rest at the pavilion. Delighted to meet a fellow student, believing Yingtai to be a man, the two scholars undertake a ritual to become blood brothers and support each other throughout their studies.

The two scholars live and study together for three years before a letter from home arrives for Yingtai asking her to return. Reluctantly she prepares to leave. She confesses to the school's mistress that she is actually a girl and in love with Shanbo. She gives the mistress a jade ornament and asks her to pass it to Shanbo as a token of love and promise of marriage. When Shanbo hears of her departure, he decides to accompany Yingtai part of the way home. On this journey, Yingtai tries to give him hints that she is really a girl. She speaks in riddles, indirectly. But Shanbo is naïve and unaware and doesn't understand her references (she is the better scholar). Finally, Yingtai says she has a younger sister and suggests that Shanbo visit, when his studies are finished, to marry her. The sister is alike in all ways, manner and voice to Yingtai so he will certainly like her.

When Yingtai arrives home, she discovers that her father has tricked her home in order to marry her off to a wealthy heir named Ma. If Yingtai refuses to marry him, it will disgrace the entire family reputation. Shortly after this, Shanbo does visit, intending to propose to Yingtai's sister. When he sees Yingtai in her female attire, and realizes that his blood brother is a woman, he falls in love. But Yingtai explains he is too late – the arranged marriage is about to be celebrated and so he leaves in great sorrow and dies quickly afterward. The day of the wedding arrives and Yingtai refuses to step into the sedan chair unless the family agree to stop the wedding parade at Shanbo's tomb on the way. She puts on a white funeral robe over her red wedding gown. At the tomb, she kneels down and sings of her love for Shanbo when suddenly a lightning bolt rends

Excavation One - deception

In pairs, read the text excerpt below in which Yingtai tries to hint that she is female. Underline the different ways Yingtai tries to reveal her gender. Discuss why Liang doesn't get it.

In the same pairs, create a scene where the two travellers have just met, and one is in disguise. Invent three riddles to give clues as to a real identity and work out some stage actions to accompany them. Perform to another pair and give each other critique. How effective or revealing is the riddle/disguise? Does the audience know more than the character and how does this affect the audience response?

Excerpt:

SHANBO: (sings) Younger brother, we have studied together for three whole years.
I suddenly find a trace of earrings on your ears;
Only women have earrings.
Younger brother, why are your ears pierced?

YINGTAI: (sings) Shanbo, you are absentminded.
Stop staring at me!
My pierced ears have a ridiculous reason –
There's a temple fair every year in my village,
And as a young boy, I was chosen to dress up like the goddess Guanyin,
So, I had to get my ears pierced.

SHANBO: Ah!

. . .

YINGTAI: (sings) Out of the city we go and over the mountain pass.
I spy a woodcutter chopping down
Firewood on top of the hill.

SHANBO: (sings) He rises early and falls into bed at night.
Gathering wood for a living is so difficult.

YINGTAI: (sings) I wonder who he does it for?

SHANBO: (sings) For his wife, of course.
Here we are at Phoenix mountain. (The phoenix is a symbol of harmony and union.)

YINGTAI: (sings) So many varied and beautiful flowers blossom here.

SHANBO: (sings) Alas, I do not see any peonies. (Symbol of romance, marriage, love.)

YINGTAI: (sings) There are some wonderful peonies at my house.
Why don't you visit me and pluck one?

SHANBO: (sings) Your peonies might be special, but I can't pluck one here and now.

YINGTAI: (sings) The green willows fall by the clear pond.
I see Mandarin ducks in couples. (Symbol of eternal love.)
Shanbo, if I were a girl,
Would you like to marry me?

SHANBO: (sings) Marry? Marry?
It's a pity that you're not a girl.

YINGTAI: (sings) We have arrived at a riverside.

SHANBO: (sings) I see a pair of white geese flying towards us. (Symbol of eternal love.)

YINGTAI: (sings) The one in front is male; the female flying behind calls him 'brother'.
You're such a goose!
It's a pity you are so thick!

SHANBO: (sings) If you think I'm thick, I won't let you call me brother anymore.

YINGTAI: (sings) A wooden bridge appears before me.
(speaks) Shanbo!
(sings) I'm scared.

SHANBO: (sings) Let me help you across.
YINGTAI: (sings) Look, there is a well. How deep is it?
I see two reflections at the bottom of the well.
A boy and a girl, smiling happily.
SHANBO: (sings) I am a boy; how dare you say I'm a girl?
We have arrived at the temple.
There's the goddess Guanyin, who brings children into the world.
YINGTAI: (sings) Guanyin is also a matchmaker.
Come on, let's get married here.
SHANBO: (sings) I'm confused.
How can two men marry?
YINGTAI: (sings) Look! Here comes a cow!
YINGTAI: (sings) What a pity Shanbo is so foolish, like a cow.
SHANBO: (sings) You really make me angry,
You can't compare me to a cow.
YINGTAI: Shanbo,
(sings) I would like to take back what I said.
Don't be angry.
(adapted by Riley)

Excavation Two – riddles in the landscape

In the same pairs, create a scene for your piece. It could be the countryside or a city landscape, but it must be packed with rich detail about the objects surrounding you, the time of day, the season, the weather, any wildlife or other actions happening around you. A common device in Chinese theatre (as in Shakespeare) is to have the actor describe the setting rather than build a realistic setting from scenery. Moreover, in Chinese theatre, the poetic description of the setting also reflects the emotions of the character speaking. The technique is called, 'borrowing from the landscape to describe feelings'. You must now build the description of the scenery into your riddle scene, making sure the landscape reflects the emotions of the piece.

The poetic, spoken environment or setting that reveals emotion may also include hints about the disguised identity. What analogies or clues might one character give to another to disguise and reveal their identity by referring to the surroundings? How can it be done subtly without giving too much away?

Excavation Three – riddles online

In a contemporary setting of the play, the actor might choose to disguise identity by assuming an online identity (catfishing). In pairs, present: a short 2-minute piece developed from the idea of online chatting. The piece must include landscape (rural or urban) that reflects feelings as well as subtle verbal and visual clues. The theatre is a place of action and embodiment, rather than reading from a screen, which is passive. How will these digital text messages appear on stage? How will you make sure the scene has live action so that it engages the audience?

Excavation Four – all-female troupes

Choose one of the contemporary all-female ensembles from Table 5.4 and after researching online, summarize, compare and discuss their mission, players, repertoire, performance sites, reviews and audience responses.

Table 5.4 Contemporary female ensembles

Arethusa Speaks	LezCab	The Queen's Company
Estrogenius Festival	Manhattan Shakespeare Project	The Radium Girls
The Dark Lady Players	Me and She Productions	Spicy Witch Company
Exquisite Corpse Company	New Georges	Teatro Luna
FAB Women (For, About and By Women)	Nora's Playhouse	The Tempest Ladies

the sky and the tomb slices open. She steps inside the tomb; it closes, and she is gone. The sky lightens, a rainbow appears, and two butterflies are seen dancing in the breeze.

In conclusion, whole-class reckoning

The impact of 'double disguise' and suspension of audience disbelief: the Yueju play is performed by an all-female cast which means that Liang Shanbo is played by a female actor playing a male and Zhu Yingtai is a female actor playing a female playing a male.

Compare this double disguise to the double disguise in As You Like it in Chapter 4, where a boy actor plays Rosalind disguised as a man pretending to be a woman.

Resources, Yueju

Goodman, Bryna and Wendy Larson. *Gender in Motion: Divisions of Labour and Cultural Change in Late Imperial and Modern China.* Lanham, MD: Rowman and Littlefield, 2005.

Jin, Jiang. *Women Playing Men: Yue Opera and Social Change in Twentieth Century Shanghai.* Seattle: University of Washington Press, 2008.

"Liang Shanbo and Zhu Yingtai." 18 October 2013. April 2020. <https://youtu.be/oJgaaGen1mA>.

Liang Shanbo and Zhu Yingtai. Dir. Sha Huang. Perf. Yuan Xuefen Fan Ruijuan. 1954. DVD.

The Lovers. Dir. Tsui Hark. Perf. Charlie Yeung Nicky Wu. 1994. DVD.

Lu, Shijun and Yilong Gao. *Think More on Producing Masterpieces and Push Yue Opera Reform.* Beijing: Zhongguo chubanshe, 1994.

Wu, Zhanfen, ed. *Fan Ruijuan biaoyan yishu The Art of Fan Ruijuan.* Shanghai: Shanghai wenyi chubanshe, 1989.

Yuan, Xuefen. *Yuan Xuefen zishu.* Shanghai: Shanghai zishu chubanshe, 2002.

CHAPTER 6

Without gender – the body

The ancient Chinese stage is roughly 7 m^2 in area and open on at least three sides. In rehearsals, the performers mentally divide the stage area into a tic-tac-toe grid of nine rectangles additionally intersected by lines dividing the stage in half vertically, horizontally and diagonally. The nine points of intersection create the best places to 'pause for a pose'. My master at the Drama Academy told me there was once a female actor who was completely blind, but she could still perform on any stage because she always knew where she and other actors were at any given moment. The only place to enter is upstage right, and the only place to exit is upstage left. So, the stage is rather like a time machine where the actor enters, completes actions and then leaves. There is no sense of an imagined bedroom or kitchen beyond the wings. An actor will enter, declare they are leaving for the palace, exit and then re-enter from the correct upstage entrance point, stating they have arrived at the palace. The stage gridlines, highly mathematical and rigid in terms of how to move in the space, are extremely helpful if you are learning how to use weapons on stage.

I am a very shy person, not a performer at all, and the only reason I went to the theatre academy in China was to find out about a different kind of theatre. Master Ma handed me a lance. First lesson in weapons training: different grips; different spinning routines; making sure the circles of the lance are in the correct axes to the floor and space around me; checking the angles of the lance in the space and against my curved arm, against a raised leg, against my back, over my head. The conventions of using the lance are strict. So much so that I could learn an entire battle choreography alone and then simply battle with another student with no need for rehearsal beforehand. I knew where my lance should be at every moment and my opponents knew their positions, so our lances and limbs met with architectural accuracy. From working with one lance, I graduated to double lance; single and double flat curved knives, or cutlasses; single and double sword; and hand-to-hand combat. The conventions pushed me into shapes and lines that were powerfully circular, robustly founded on foot and hip position with the curving line from shoulder to wrist tightly controlled. There are differences in playing male and female warrior – shifts in the balance of a knee, the circumference of arms, the tilt of the head – but this was my first exposure to feeling in control of a completely 3D space. I could slice it, embrace it, sweep it with my weapons – the battle sequences held me confident and empowered. As a

DOI: 10.4324/9781003080800-7

European, I doubt any other activity on stage could have given me this sense of strength and control.

The conventions I learned through weapons training for the stage in China taught me that the body can be deceived. The body can learn, adopt and modify patterns of movement that make you feel very different from your usual self. By shifting the physical pattern of your body – the way you always move, stand and walk – you can explore different emotions and ideas of yourself. You can be another body.

Performance of chance - Merce Cunningham

'Overthrow the notion of the narrative . . . movement itself becomes the narrative' (Walker Arts Center). Merce Cunningham (1919–2009), dancer and choreographer, felt that story could be found in many different places. His work became increasingly abstract, making the audience work to create meaning rather than being offered a complete piece with a narrative beginning, middle and end. Cunningham's aim was to get rid of cliché and celebrate unexpected moments of collision, deviation and idiosyncrasy. A performance was not considered finished, or even the same, each night. As a dancer/choreographer, Cunningham and musician John Cage (composer) experimented with the idea that a performance might be made up of different elements that have no intentional connection with each other, but which nonetheless create myriads of meaning in the mind's eye of the spectator. Cunningham said 'The mind gets in the way' (Walker Arts Center), meaning chance operations would help to eliminate his own innate bias and choices in structuring his work. For example, Cunningham and Cage separately created a work of a fixed duration before putting the two pieces together for the first time on stage. The result was a movement piece that had no obvious link to the musical soundscape. The same technique was used with artists such as Robert Rauschenberg, Jasper Johns and Andy Warhol, who produced art works for the stage that were seen for the first time by the performers when they appeared on stage to perform, 'i asked RobERt RausChenbeRg to mAkE somEthiNg FOr It. tHe dAnCe wAs not FiNisHed. i did nOt tell Him what to mAke, only tHat it Could be sOmetHing That wAs In thE dANCe area, that wE could Move ThroUgh it, ArounD it, anD with iT if He so LikED' (Cunningham, Changes: Notes on Choreography).

While actual movement phrases were carefully composed in advance, Merce Cunningham and John Cage looked to flipping coins, the Chinese I-Ching with its 8 trigrams and 64 possible combinations; throwing a dice and computer-generated random numbers to make choices about the timing, duration and number of dancers for movements. Cunningham felt that randomly chosen operations would create moments he could not have conceived of by himself, that they 'opened up a new facet of a new possibility' (Walker Arts Center). In fact, both artists looked to Eastern philosophy to inspire their work, not just by consulting the I-Ching but also Buddhism. John Cage recounts that Buddha was asked how to become enlightened and answered, 'it comes gradually . . . like the germination of seeds and . . . it comes suddenly . . . like lightning and thunder' (Walker Arts Center). The paradox of how enlightenment happens is not unlike the paradox of the work Cunningham and Cage were producing. Cunningham would compose a stream of movements or phrases and then use chance to structure them together. He also broke the limitations of a theatre stage by performing outside in stone quarries, on beaches, in sculpture gardens, a circus arena and in museums (Walker Arts Center). Cage said that if you want to see art, just sit on a bench in a park and put a frame around what you see. Your intention (your chosen framing) makes it art.

Process over product

Cunningham was fascinated by and loved to manipulate all kinds of technology. He used the camera as an actor on stage moving in and out of the action to show different perspectives of the action. He also celebrated the camera's ability to focus on a small detail of action or body and thus shift the sense of scale and proportion as he was interested in the individual body parts that might operate independently of each other. He used intercut scenes and cuts in general to break up the flow of a sequence randomly and shift tempo unexpectedly.

So random

Cunningham and Cage had a fascination with time and felt that it was up to the spectator to determine what the piece was 'about'. A performance was created by the simple, simultaneous presence of people moving, people playing music, people creating art works, people listening and people watching within a specified timeframe. When the curtain comes down, the performance is at an end. The curtain falls at a specific time, agreed in advance, rather than when a planned movement piece has reached its culmination. Cunningham firmly believed in the momentariness of a performance. Unlike a painting, a musical score, a play-text or a poem, there is no artefact that remains after the performance is over. For Cunningham there is only the fleeting moment that has been experienced by those present, which includes all artists and spectators in that moment of time in that space.

> *In Space, the dancers had possibilities for improvisation within a space scale. . . . My original idea for the costumes was that they be picked up or found in the particular playing situation we were in, and that the set or the way the stage looked would also be devised from the existing circumstances and environment at the time of the performance. The title does not refER TO ANY IMPLICIT OR EXPLICIT NARRATIVE BUT TO THE FACT THAT EVERY SPECTATOR MAY SEE AND HEAR THE EVENTS IN THEIR OWN WAY. WITHIN A SECTION THE MOVEMENTS GIVEN TO A PARTICULAR DANCER COULD CHANGE IN SPACE AND TIME AND THE ORDER THE DANCER CHOSE TO DO THEM IN COULD COME FROM THE INSTANT OF DOING THEM. ALSO, THE LENGTH OF EACH SECTION VARIED EACH TIME.* (Cunningham, Changes: Notes on Choreography)

Circles

Merce Cunningham created a piece called 'Ocean', that premièred at the Cirque Royale in Brussels in 1994 (Ocean). The circular arena allowed him to play with the 64 hexagrams of the I-Ching, doubled to make 128, for the sake of lengthening the performance. The circular space prevented the performers from feeling there was a 'front'. Everywhere was 'front'. This was not a new concept for Cunningham and his dancers, but it gave physical shape to their established aesthetic. Cunningham told his performers it would be like dancing on a moving carousel.

Any work of Merce Cunningham has reverberations and resonations of the various artists that inspired him. These included people like John Cage, Andy Warhol, Robert Rauschenberg, Roy Lichtenstein, Jasper Johns. John Cage was inspired by a comment made by a literature professor about the work of novelist James Joyce, who increasingly used a technique aimed to recreate dreams and the subconscious. Joyce's book, *Finnegans Wake*, for example, is written in a blend of puns, stream of consciousness, literary allusions, associations and many different languages. Its cyclical structure begins and ends like this:

> riverrun, past Eve and Adams, from swerve of shore to bend of bay, brings us by a commodius vicus of recirculation back to Howth, Castle and Environs.
>
> Sir Tristram, violer d'amores, fr'over the short sea, had passencore rearrived from North Armorica on this side the scraggy isthmus of Europe Minor to wielderfight his penisolate war; nor had topsawyer's rocks by the stream Oconee exaggerated themselse to Laurens County's giorgios while they went doublin their mumper all the time. . . . (Joyce 3)

Cage and Cunningham's good friend and literary scholar, Joseph Campbell, predicted Joyce's next work might be about water. This was the starting point for Ocean, alongside John Cage's dream of performing 'in the round'. What's important here is that Cunningham did not work in isolation but drew his inspiration and creativity from many other artists and art forms.

Contemporary dancer, Siobhan Davies, developed a similar idea of circularity and repetition in her piece, 'The Score' (Davies). Watch excerpts from both these pieces, Ocean and The Score online, to see how the circular shape of the performance area challenges and inspires the movements on stage.

Excavation One – walking

Watch Merce Cunningham's piece BIPED 1999.

'In the case of humans, you have two feet which carry you around and they, to me, are the source of all movement. It doesn't mean you always have to use them, there are other possibilities, but the legs are a principal way of moving around and getting from one place to another. There is a very simple basic thing about the basic thing of moving when you walk. What do you do? You move all right, step out to someplace but in the course of stepping you have to close your feet as you change from one step to another which brings about everything else' (Walker Arts Center).

In pairs, explore walking in all its forms. Break down the movement of the sole of the foot, the ball of the foot, and the toes, the ankles, the position of the hips, torso, shoulders and head, arms, fingers. Explore speeds, rhythms, size of steps. Explore walking with intention towards different goals, explore walking with no goal. Explore walking towards each other and away from each other. Create a film sequence of walking, including different kinds of walk in barefoot, in boots, in socks, in shoes, in heels. Include close-up shots of the foot and steps as well as wide shots of the whole body. Intercut with any other video footage you find on your phone and add a randomly chosen piece of music.

Survey the terrain

To walk is to move; to move is to dance.

Excavation Two – walking the circle

Browse the two performances online: Cunningham's Ocean and Davies The Score (see resources below).

In a group of four to five, discuss how you could create your own pathways on a circular stage with no 'front'. What might inspire your circular idea? Thought-shower some ideas with your group. Will your circular space indicate a clock, planet, ball, round fruit, dinner plate, pizza, cake, wheel, number 0, letter O, clown's nose, fried egg, or coin, for example?

What patterns or divisions or intersections of your circular performance space make sense to your concept (a circle within a circle for the fried egg, for example). What kinds of movement might be appropriate?

Mark your dissection lines as a group by walking them, remembering some of the walking explorations from excavation 1.

Once a basic structure and movement is in place, decide on a randomization process such as a dice, a spinner, pulling straws, an online randomization programme, to allow you to change while performing:

- **The speed** of movements: tempo, direction, intensity, number of walkers
- **The duration** of movements: pause, unison, anchor, direction, dissolve, repeat, rewind, pulse, compress, expand.
- **The weight** of movements: heavy, light, flicking, slapping, floating, sinking, stamping, tiptoeing.
- **The spatial perspective** of movements: foreground/background, convergence/divergence, facing, balance, collapse, rise.
- **The shape** of movements: curved, symmetrical, diagonal, angular, open, closed, tense, loose, heavy/light, sudden/slow, high/low.

Now add a soundtrack by taking any middle sections from six random of tracks in your music library and cutting them together without planning. The resulting track must be at least 90 seconds long. Put the performance together with the music. It might complement, jar against, emphasize or destroy your spatial idea.

Setting the compass

The randomization of moves nonetheless generates meaning in the minds of those who are watching.

Excavation Three – the dice

Depending on the age of the students, either select six everyday actions, such as brushing teeth, running for the bus, turning the page of a book, or provide six movements from the Laban basic movements (Newlove and Dalby). List them, allocating each movement sequence or style a number from 1 to 6.

In pairs, take a dice and throw once. You must execute the movement sequence/movement indicated on your list by the numbers you throw in any way you choose.

Now throw twice more to make three moves in total and fix these movements by repeating them.

Now consider transitions between each movement. Think about the way you interact as pairs: you can move identically (unison); in mirror formation (opposition); in front and behind each other; in syncopated movement; one after the other, touching each other, not touching each other, close to each other, at a distance from each other, shadowing, meeting, parting, copying, solo, canon, scattering, gathering.

Now pair up with another pair to make a group of four and teach each other your sequences to make one longer sequence that includes all six moves and transitions with all four people.

Choose and agree to a specific performance space and be conscious of where the audience will be located.

Prepare the piece in the chosen space. Each group chooses a soundscape or piece of music. You will play your group's soundscape or music for different group, however. They will not know what it is until they start to perform!

Excavation Four – the cinematic eye

Some members of the class volunteer to act as camera operators. In pairs, using phones, your job is to capture the movement piece of one group in a series of clips. You can move in and out of the piece; you can focus on a small area or part of the body; you can keep the camera still. Each recorded clip should be no longer than 3 seconds. Once you have generated enough material, you may also leave the rehearsal space and film anything you see outside the studio to intercut with the movement sequence that might support, jar, contrast, lift your sequence. Remove all sound. Edit all your filmed material together to create one sequence, including both movement and the random footage from outside the studio. You do not need to follow the chronology of the original sequence. You are making your own 'movement sequence' from the images. Once the sequence is edited to your satisfaction, add the soundtrack provided by another group. Share films.

Resetting the compass

Creating a movement piece that resists telling a story.
  Celebrating the unexpected 'moments' in performance.
  Which moments would one reject or do differently?
  A performance is a transient moment in time never to be repeated.

Excavation Five – 'The only way to do it, is to do it' (Walker Arts Centre)

All physical theatre and dance performers struggle to find a way to notate their creations. Although Cunningham was a firm believer in randomization, nonetheless, the movement sequences and patterns were documented throughout the creative process. One page from his notes includes the circular turns in one sequence and his comment, 'the only way to do it, is to do it' (see Figure 6.1).

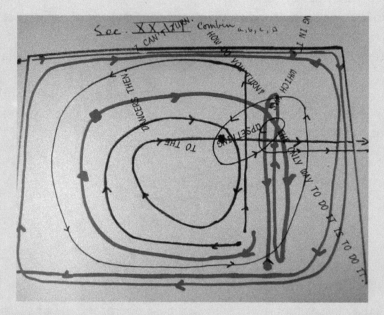

Figure 6.1 'The only way to do it, is to do it' (Cunningham, Changes) by kind permission of the Merce Cunningham Trust.

In small groups of two to three, look closely at the excerpts from Merce Cunningham's diary in Figures 6.2–6.5. The drawings were not made from real-life observations, but while on tour; Merce Cunningham liked to read nature magazines and let his thoughts and ideas wander in choosing these subjects to draw.

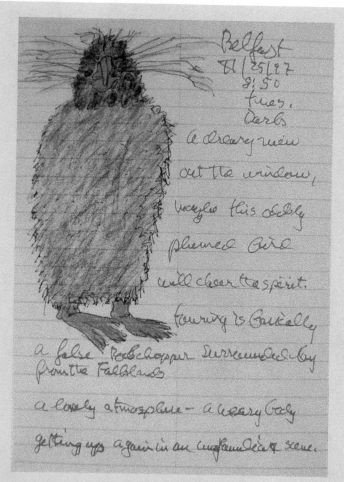

Figure 6.2 'Dark, a dreary view' (Cunningham, Other Animals 58) by kind permission of the Merce Cunningham Trust.

Belfast XI/25/97 8.50 Tues
Dark
a dreary view out the window,
maybe this oddly plumed bird
will cheer the spirit.
touring is basically
a false rockhopper
from the Falklands
surrounded by a lonely atmosphere etc – a heavy body
getting up again in an unfamiliar scene

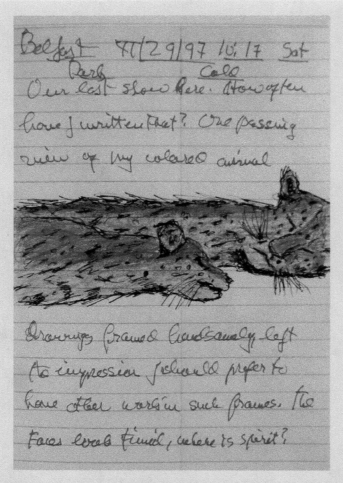

Figure 6.3 'Our last show here' (Cunningham, Other Animals 59) by kind permission of the Merce Cunningham Trust.

Belfast XI/29/97 10:17 Sat
> Dark Cold
> Our last show here. How often
> have I written that? One passing
> view of my colored animal
> drawings framed handsomely, left
> an impression I should prefer to
> have other works in such frames. The faces look timid, where is the spirit?

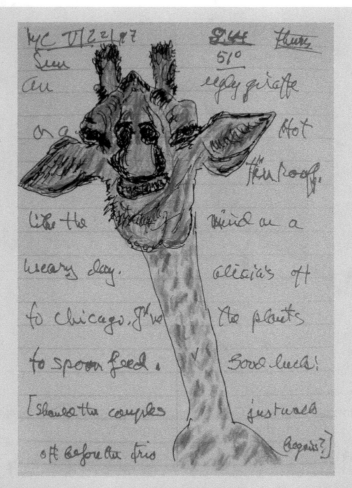

Figure 6.4 'Should the couples just walk off?' (Cunningham, Other Animals 52) by kind permission of the Merce Cunningham Trust.

NYC V/22/97 8.44 Thursday
 Sun 51°
 An ugly giraffe
 on a hot
 tin roof.
 like the mind on a
 weary day. Alicia's off
 to Chicago. I've the plants
 to spoon feed. Good luck!
 (should the couples just walk
 off before the trio begins?)

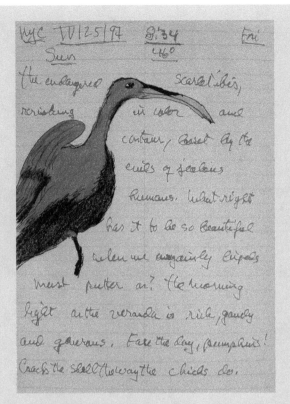

Figure 6.5 'We ungainly bipeds' (Cunningham, Other Animals 42) by kind permission of the Merce Cunningham Trust.

NYC IV/25/97 8.34 Fri
  Sun 46°
  The endangered scarlet ibis,
  resisting in colour and
  contour, beset by the
  evils of jealous
  humans. What right
  has it to be so beautiful
  when we ungainly bipeds
  must putter on? The morning
  light on the veranda is rich, gaudy
  and glorious. Face the day pumpkins!
  (Cunningham, Merce Cunningham and Other Animals 42-59)

The words and images from Merce Cunningham's diary seem to be randomly collated on each page. There is a drawing from something in a magazine, notes on the date, the weather and time, as well as emotions, feelings, moods and instructions about the household and notes for the dancers at the evening's performance. Each page captures some disparate and random thoughts from a slice of time.

Discuss the words and images on one of the pages with a partner. Over the next 48 hours, each student should record – in sketches, words, phrases, clippings, photos – any random ideas, thoughts, events, objects they find interesting. Note, in particular, things that move.

Return to the studio and in groups of four to five share the 48-hour journal pages with the group. As an example of the give-and-take of building a piece with another artist in a collaborative way, see how, very early in their collaboration, John Cage writes about composing music for Cunningham's ideas. Cage said,

> The scenario given me . . . 'the fullness of a Summer's day' suggested that Summer would be the longest section; that, together with his desire that each season would be developed by continuous invention and preceded by a short prelude . . . and that the entire work would be cyclical and concise, brought about the following numerical situation: 2,2; 1,3; 2,4; 1,3; 1. . . . (Cunningham, Changes: Notes on Choreography)

Add any comments or sticky notes to each other's drawings, noting associations, commentaries, inspirations and interpretations that arise from reading each other's work.

Each student selects one or two moments from the collaborative journal their group has compiled and works on physicalizing them in one or two simple moves: for example, the stance of the ibis, shifting from foot to foot or a 'heavy body getting up'. Teach all moves to each other in the group.

Plot the space by mapping a chosen mathematical figure to the studio floor. Mark each point where each of the moves rehearsed above could take place and allocate each space a phrase or word belonging to the move from the collaborative journal. Use an online text randomizer or scissors and glue to shuffle the lines in different ways for each member of the group. Perform!

Alternatively, allocate a number from 1 to 6 to each performance space and have students toss the dice to determine individual sequences.

Remember, there is no rehearsal, no preparation; just do it! Allow for pause if someone is using the space required; allow for collisions or collusions, if it so happens.

Whole-class reckoning

'The only way to do it, is to do it'.

Excavation Six – falling is also moving

In 1997, Merce Cunningham worked with media developer, Paul Kaiser, on the piece Hand Drawn Spaces. The aim was to integrate 3D and 2D bodies virtually and live on stage, which Kaiser felt was a way to show the inside workings of Cunningham's mind. A device Kaiser used was 'to construct metaphorical mental spaces . . . to create worlds that depicted how their minds worked' (Kaiser).

Individually, each student reviews the key ideas, images, text pieces or movement ideas from their personal 48-hour journal. Create a sequence of six moves with or without text that demonstrate the actual writing or drawing of some elements of the journal. The moves could be expanded, exaggerated, reduced, distorted, contorted, fragmented – they do not need to be realistic. Kaiser comments: 'I was always very interested in drawing, even from my work with kids. What struck me about the way that kids draw is that the drawings are more interesting as performance than they are as a finished art product. What you see on your refrigerator door doesn't tell you as much as if you were watching the kid make the drawing'. So, the movement sequence should be composed of the movements of actually drawing/writing in the journal. It is not a representation of what the artist has drawn in the journal. It is a movement sequence that describes the hand as it writes or draws the inner workings of the mind.

A similar process is seen in Indonesian shadow puppet theatre, Wayang Orang, where actors imitate the puppet shadow movements from Wayang Kulit shadow puppet performances. That is, the actors imitate the shadows of the shadow puppets and puppeteers.

Bearing in mind the sequence of thoughts in movement, choose a relevant performance space and define the performance area: for example, perhaps the surface of two steps in a flight of six; a table top and underneath the table; a circular spiral around an object; a starburst from an object. The performance space should topographically represent the inner image of each student's individual mind. Combine to make a group of three or five and organize the space so that all can work in the same general area even if there are overlaps and collisions between each student's performance mind space. With no forward planning, the group share their representations of the individual inner minds.

To both of these randomized performances, add battery-operated bicycle headlights (they can change colour and flash); add reflector strips on the body. Cunningham stated, 'the lighting is done freely each time, differently, so that the RHYTHMS OF THE MOVEMENTS are differently accented and the shapes differently seen, partially or not at all' (Cunningham, Changes: Notes on Choreography).

Add random music (without lyrics); atmosphere soundtrack; have performers wear light-coloured clothing and project moving images onto them; set up a live stream and project onto the performance area simultaneously; add a significant prop each; play with stage lights or any other production element. Share and reflect.

Whole-class reckoning

'Falling is also moving'.

Resources, Merce Cunningham

"BIPED." 25 October 2016. *YouTube*. March 2020. <https://youtu.be/QetwaIcxaiM>.

Cunningham, Merce. *Changes: Notes on Choreography*. Ed. The Merce Cunningham Trust. New York: The Song Cave and Merce Cunningham Trust, 2019.

—. *Merce Cunningham and Other Animals*. New York: Aperture, 2002.

Davies, Siobhan. "The Score." April 2020. *Siobhandavies.com*. March 2020. <https://youtu.be/0c67d0o_WT8>.

Joyce, James. *Finnegans Wake*. Wordsworth, 2012.

Kaiser, Paul. "Hand Drawn Spaces." 2019. *Open-Ended Group*. March 2020. <https://player.vimeo.com/video/32776116?title=0&byline=0&portrait=0>.

Newlove, Jean and John Dalby. *Laban for All*. Nick Hern Books, 2003.

"Ocean." 7 August 2009. *YouTube*. March 2020. <https://youtu.be/1aBJdHnv5tM>.

Walker Arts Center. *Chance Conversations – An Interview with Merce Cunningham and John Cage*. 27 July 2009. 28 February 2020. <https://www.youtube.com/watch?v=ZNGpjXZovgk>.

—. *Merce Cunningham's Working Process*. 28 July 2009. February 2020. <https://www.youtube.com/watch?v=zhK3Ep4Hil0>.

—. *The Six Sides of Merce Cunningham*. 22 February 2017. 28 February 2020. <https://www.youtube.com/watch?v=xJeum_kxSV8>.

Interactive projection performance - Robert Lepage

Robert Lepage (b1957) graduated from Quebec City Conservatoire d'Art Dramatique, and studied in Paris with Alain Knapp, who championed the idea that the creative experience was only possible if the actors, writers, directors and designers were equal collaborators. Knapp demanded that the actor is part of the creative work, not merely an interpreter of a given text (Bunzil). Later, Lepage worked in Quebec at the Théâtre Repère with the director Jacques Lessard, who created a recipe for creating theatre: Resources, Score, Valuaction and Performance, RSVP:

R = Resources: the human and physical resources at your disposal.

S = Scores which describe the process leading to the performance.

V = Valuaction that looks at the results of action, selecting and dumping ideas as well as decision-making.

P = Process which is the end result of scores and represents the style of the process.

Designed for use in urban planning and architecture, the RSVP system was developed earlier by dancer Anna Halprin and her architect husband Lawrence, in the 1960s. The cycle was supposed to show that the apparent end of the process is only the beginning of a new process. Performance is in a perpetual process of change and renewal with work beginning from any point within the creative cycle (Dundjerovic 30). Anna Halprin also strove to move the passive spectator into an active participant. The performance was only 'scored' or outlined, and much was left open, so that the piece emerged according to the interactions between performer and audience in a specific moment of time, never to be repeated or captured. The pieces were highly collaborative and included dancers, visual artists, designers, psychologists, writers, musicians and teachers (Hirsch). Here are all the elements of Lepage's later highly collaborative work and echoes of the practice of Merce Cunningham.

Robert Lepage creates performances that evolve from a lengthy process of discovery and rehearsal. The play is not 'finished' until its very last performance, just as each performance is changed by each audience resulting in different interactions between actors and audience in the moment. These can be significant changes of structure, flow and even entire scenes. The rehearsal period is long, with breaks of weeks and months, sometimes years, in between to allow for the subconscious mind of the performer to build and change ideas. The mind is like is an active subconscious which Lepage calls a 'rendering farm'. During rehearsals, he measures the length of a potential piece by comparing it to the gestation period of an animal. Is it a 'hamster' – 22 days; a dog – 9 weeks; a human – 9 months; or an elephant – 24 months? (Banff Centre for Arts and Creativity). Lepage's productions often have multiple plotlines and layers of meaning, large casts, vast sets and intensive technical input. The productions are generally in 'long form' and can last up to 11 hours, with breaks. Lepage also invites the audience to attend rehearsals and give feedback which is then fed into the continuing creative process. He compares the rehearsal process to a journey by Christopher Columbus since the company knows they are heading for a continent, but they don't know yet what the shape of it might be. The only people that can help the Lepage ensemble shape it is the audience itself (Banff Centre for Arts and Creativity).

The RSVP system

Resource: Lepage prefers to start the work from a resource, an actual object, rather than a theme. The resource should have a personal resonance to the actor who offers it. Stories, dreams, anecdotes and myths can be resources. It is something solid that may then lead to an emotion or idea. For Lepage it is easier to start an improvisation from a torn letter than the theme of broken love (Dundjerovic 84) because tearing paper is an action, not an abstract idea. The essence of theatre is action.

Score: the score is an event that occurs, a fragment of an action, with its own narrative. Each actor-writer will develop a score in their own way. A score may be a written or drawn account of the moment, showing floor movement, space, action, sound, and it may be complete or open. Shakespeare's scores were open, in that he mostly only recorded exits and entrances, for example. Lepage prefers open scores (not unlike the Commedia dell'arte scenarios). The performance is the moment where the various scores might collide, juxtapose, underscore each other and create meaning in the spectator's mind.

Valuaction: after each exploration, during each exploration moment, there is an evaluating process held by all the theatre makers involved – designers, actors, musicians and technical crew. These reflective evaluations become decisions about what to what to get rid of, what to keep, what to keep changing and trying.

Triggers

The theatre of Robert Lepage is intensely visual, and his use of projections highlights this. However, he denies the visual aspect is the most important, since he feels that the images he chooses are mere 'triggers' for the audience from which to make their own visual constructions. Lepage insists that radio is the ultimate visual medium, since it requires the listeners to create images in their imaginations. Sometimes the voice acts as a soundscape, or modulations of sound, rather than actual words. Lepage views voice as a vehicle that generates resonance, echo and response (Theater Museum Canada), and many of his productions have been more opera than plays, 'Is it music sound or noise? I like that to be blurred' (The Soundpeople). The voice, soundscape and music flow naturally from Lepage's fascination with different spoken languages and ways of speaking. Lepage grew up bilingual French and English and also speaks Spanish, Italian, Japanese, German and Swedish. Sound fulfils Lepage's aim to make the audience 'work' to participate in creating a performance in their minds and imaginations alongside the actors on stage. Sound is a trigger to something more. In the same way, Lepage draws audience attention away from 'what does the playwright mean' to finding triggers in the choreography, gesture, soundscape and music as well (The Soundpeople). The creative process in building a performance is of key importance to Lepage. Sometimes, however, creative decisions are driven by purely technical motives. Lepage believes Shakespeare included so many soliloquies in Hamlet, primarily as a practical consideration to allow the other actors time to change costume off stage between scenes. Thus, for Lepage, any problems that he encounters in creating the piece are always primarily connected to technical, staging solutions (Banff Centre for Arts and Creativity).

Synthesis of art forms

Lepage regards theatre as a synthesis of equally important, but different, art forms such as painting, music and sculpture, for example, not unlike Wagner's concept of the Gesamtkunstwerk. Consequently, Lepage also explores digital projection and interactive projection as an equal 'actor' in the performance, and actor and technology evolve together as 'writing-in-performance'. Lepage considers the performance like a 'score'. By this, he means the vertical mapping of different art forms that connect to each other at any one given moment. Rather than having a playtext, or director's book and designer's portfolio, the performance is notated as simultaneous, multilayered moments of performance and production elements on one page. A performance is only one 'reading' out of the many possible readings other performances may provoke, just as one orchestra's performance of a concerto will differ each night, though each instrumentalist and the conductor are working from one 'score'.

Techno en scène

A key actor in a Lepage production is recorded visual and/or sound material. Despite enormous budgets, the production techniques are actually quite straightforward and 'low tech', almost 'poor theatre'. Techno en scène is a term used to describe the combination and interaction of technology with human actors on stage just as mise en scène describes the interaction of the set with the human actors. Techno en scène combines live performance with video, slide projections, digital technologies, sound recordings and cinematic imagery (Dundjerovic 181). Digital technology can transform space and time making the theatre seem transformative and flexible, never fixed, thus reflecting the creative process of the human actors.

Décalage - jet lag

Lepage uses the term décalage which in modern French means 'jet-lag', a sense of dislocation, both mental and physical disorientation. Lepage uses the term as 'discrepancy' in time – like being in two or more places at once, two or more times at once and feeling 'at home' or comfortable in either. Décalage refers to the multi-lingual, multi-cultured being who is nowhere at home and always a visitor. In his work, décalage means acknowledging the gaps between things, allowing things to be 'fuzzy' or difficult to determine. The creative energy is built on impulse and intuition that can create simultaneity and juxtaposition or contrast. The actor, projection text, object, sound and audience are pulled into a dialogue, questioning and reacting to each other in an active way as they 'build' the performance together. There is no linear development of a story but multiple stories that are fragmented and overlaid with each other. Lepage uses filmic devices such as close-ups and intercuts, or montage, to highlight and exaggerate specific moments; to juxtapose contrasting moments, to jump between scenes. In his production of the 7 Streams of the River Ota, all the occupants of a New York tenement are in the bathroom at the same time without seeing each other (Bunzil).

Framing

The theatre provides a frame or viewpoint which can focus or draw attention to one or other of the various art forms working together. Lepage's role as a director is to hold up that frame – whether it is a light, a projection, a gesture, a word or piece of music in order to highlight a specific moment. Lepage suggests a frame can be like a stethoscope that fixates spectator attention on the particular heartbeat of an action (Theater Museum Canada). One of his productions, Macbeth, consisted entirely of picture frames and the interaction of the actors with and behind and through such frames.

Communion not communication

The purpose of the performance is to join with the audience in a shared event, according to Lepage. It is not to communicate a particular meaning, statement or opinion to the audience.

Excavation One – digital impro

The aim of this exploration is to create an experience in theatre that is derived from a process of exploration of digital projection, sound, light, movement and voice and to use these elements to trigger the audience into collaborating in creating the moment.

Resource

Bring an object to class that has some kind of connection to you. Share your object with a partner. Map together what possible connections, differences, stories and ideas your two objects bring.

With your partner, take 15 minutes to film on your phone anything and everything you can find that moves, that seems like it might belong to your stories whether emotionally, or literally, through shape, colour or line. It might be hordes of children going upstairs; wind blowing through branches; cars on the street. Each clip should be no longer than 3 seconds. Bring all the clips back into the classroom and share in one folder.

In the studio, arrange a screen with projector behind, connected to the computer. Change the projection mode to back projection. One at a time, each student enters the stage in front of the screen. Play one clip on a loop, without sound, and allow the student to watch a few times. The student then turns to face the audience and improvises a moment that interacts in some way with the movement of objects on the screen. They can imitate the movements; juxtapose their movements to the screen; interact with the movements on the screen. In each case, respond immediately; adapt and modify as the loop replays; play with the image on the screen as much as you can. Let it play you. This is digital projection improvisation and the same rules of improvisation apply:

Say Yes!

There are no mistakes!

Listen, watch, respond!

All students have access to the shared folder and can use material from it at any time.

Excavation Two – scale

Now with a different partner, go out and film again. This time look at scale. Choose parts of faces that are talking, hands and feet that move, mouths, eyes, ears – choose to film close up, choose to film at a distance. Repeat the exercise from above, looping your human clips and focusing on the movement inspired by the clip in improvisation.

Excavation Three – techno en scène

You will need to experiment with projectors, cables, computers, your phones and cameras. You need to learn how to connect the cables and connect to sound if needed. Consider the positioning of screens or use white sheets draped over objects to create a 3D screen shape; white costuming; multiple projection areas. Play with the technology and see what it can do for you. Livestream is easy to create with an old-fashioned digital video camcorder cabled into the projector, or your phone to computer to projector. Use the livestream to focus in, zoom out, pan, tilt, be part of the action on stage while your vision of it is simultaneously projected onto a chosen part of the stage. See what happens when . . .

Excavation Four – score

With your partner, join with another pair to make a group of four. Can the four stories derived from your four original resources be intertwined, connected, juxtaposed, meshed? Explore practically with the projected clips/images from the shared folder.

   As you build, follow the example of Figure 6.6 to document some moments of the process of exploration.

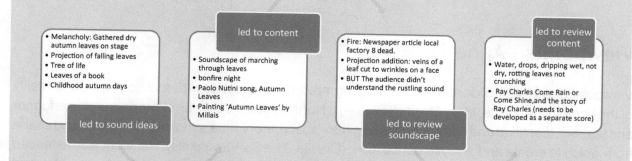

Figure 6.6 Resource: leaf progression of ideas.

Add sound, add music, add words, add costume – whatever the piece needs. If costume, then why this costume? Think period, think gender, think formal or casual, think colour, think character, think cohesive, think jarring . . .

Excavation Five – valuaction

Use coloured highlighters, underlining, arrows on your work to show which ideas to keep and which to drop. This is the valuaction part of the process – looking for actions, making decisions about what is worth keeping.

In conclusion, whole-class reckoning

Interactive projection is simply another potential collaborator in the creative theatre process.

   The interactivity of projection – not to be used as a simple backdrop – reinforces the idea of the synthesis of many different art forms coming together with an audience to create a moment of theatre.

Resources, Lepage

Banff Centre for Arts and Creativity. "Robert Lepage Creating Outside of the Frame." 14 July 2014. *YouTube.* Banff Centre Talks. 21 January 2020. <https://www.youtube.com/watch?v=pMGPzuF7B_Q>.

Bunzil, James. "The Geography of Creation: Décalage as Impulse, Process and Outcome in the Theatre of Robert Lepage." *The Drama Review* 43.1 (Spring) (1999): 79–103.

Dundjerovic, Aleksandar S. *The Theatricality of Robert Lepage.* Montreal: McGill Queen's University Press, 2007.

Hirsch, Alison B. "The Collective Creativity of Anna and Lawrence Halprin." July 2016. *Grantmakers in the Arts.* February 2020. <https://www.giarts.org/article/collective-creativity-anna-and-lawrence-halprin>.

Theater Museum Canada. "Robert Lepage on Durational Performance." 20 January 2011. *YouTube.* 23 January 2020. <https://youtu.be/layLHxPDgck>.

—. "Robert Lepage on the Visual Imagination, and Audiences Part 9/9." 20 January 2011. *YouTube.* February 17 2020. <https://youtu.be/3sZX1C4_IZU>.

—. "Robert Lepage on Voice, Speech and Lipsynch 1–9." 4 February 2011. *YouTube.* 12 February 2020. <https://youtu.be/8pT_KHH4S8g>.

The Soundpeople. "Interview with Robert Lepage." 9 September 2017. *YouTube.* February 2020. <https://www.youtube.com/watch?v=hdQIaOCxXBU>.

Viewpoints – Anne Bogart

Viewpoints is a system of describing and creating movement sequences. It is focused on the physicality of the body. In the 1970s, Mary Overlie (1946–), a North American dancer, choreographer, performer and teacher, identified and named Six Viewpoints – space, story, time, emotion, movement and shape from which to create and analyse dance work (Overlie, The Six Viewpoints). Her work was extended some years later by theatre director Anne Bogart (1951–), North American theatre director and professor at Columbia University. She founded the SITI (Saratoga International Theatre Institute), alongside Suzuki Tadashi, to revitalize contemporary theatre in the United States. Suzuki Tadashi (1939–) is a theatre director/writer who founded the theatre company SCOT (Suzuki Company of Toga) and developed an actor's training system derived extensively from traditional Japanese No theatre. His company is focused on intercultural exchange. Anne Bogart also collaborated with Tina Landau (1962–), who is a North American playwright/director focused on ensemble work and member of the Steppenwolf Theatre Company. Like Merce Cunningham and Robert Lepage and their multiple collaborations, artistic communication and exchange between a number of different artists provokes revolutionary theatre ideas. Anne Bogart and Tina Landau published their work on nine Viewpoints known simply as Viewpoints (Bogart and Landau).

Bogart's nine Viewpoints: spatial relationships, kinesthetic response, shape, gesture, repetition, architecture, tempo, duration and topography are practical in-roads to creating and devising movement pieces. Viewpoints is focused on the body in space and ensemble work. The performers rehearse in a clearly defined square space, marked as a grid, not unlike the demarcations of the traditional Japanese No and Chinese stages. This connection is likely a product of the collaboration between Anne Bogart and Suzuki Tadashi, whose system of actor training drew heavily on No actor training methods (see Chapter 5). The Viewpoints system is a practical technique for developing physicality that also addresses the aesthetics, emotions and text of a performance piece. Both Overlie and Bogart felt that performance had become too plot-focused; the story had become too important. In response, Viewpoints suggests, first, that all the performance and production elements that contribute to a piece are equally important. Second, meaning is constructed in the spectator's mind when observing the movement of bodies in space. Therefore, the performance only has meaning when the spectators are present and actively involved in the process. Buckwalter describes a performance by Mary Overlie where she enters, picks up an orange electricity cable and unwinds it as she moves around the stage. There is a socket in the back wall, and the spectators interpret the workman-like movements of Overlie with a story about construction. However, Overlie finally comes to rest with the end of the cable held up to a ladder. The spectator suddenly sees the picture made by the orange cable in space – an artwork in day-glo orange (Buckwalter 31). Viewpoints can also be used in dialogue and vocal work, writing, blocking text on stage, devising, rehearsing, music and group improvisation (Bogart and Landau). The Viewpoints system is an open process where performers are encouraged to make their own discoveries. Viewpoints should not be followed in a linear way, step by step, except in learning about them. Accidents, coincidences and happenstance are key to the process.

The Viewpoints are:

- **Spatial relationship:** the distance between things (objects, bodies etc.) onstage.
- **Kinesthetic response:** how performers respond to movement from other people, objects or design elements.
- **Shape:** the outline of a body or object in space.
- **Gesture:** a behavioural or expressive shape that has a beginning, middle and end.
- **Repetition:** when performers recreate something that they have done or seen.
- **Architecture:** a performer's physical environment.
- **Tempo:** how fast or slowly something happens onstage.
- **Duration:** how long a movement lasts in time.
- **Topography:** the onstage pattern or design a movement creates. (Bogart and Landau)

Before any explorations begin, establish a working practice that is safe: the studio is free from clutter, flooring is suitable for movement work and students are barefoot or with suitable footwear. Use trust exercises and hard physical warmups to break barriers and encourage a sense of ensemble and safe practice. Establish a contract of care.

Make sure the performers are physically warmed up and hungry to explore. Through the Body by Dymphna Callery (Callery) and Frantic Assembly have some wonderful physical exercises for warmups (Graham and Hoggett) using space and physical devising.

Excavation One – table top

As a whole-class exercise, choose any two random objects and place them on a table top. Show them to the onlookers and then stand in front of them to hide them while you change their positions. The minute the objects are (re)placed on the table the spectators create new information about them, their relationship to each other and begin to make narratives or stories about a possible sequence of events – who put them there; where is that person now; what will happen next. Demonstrate to the class that every positioning in space of every object and or body has meaning but everyone who sees it will probably deduce a different meaning – and that's exciting (Buckwalter 146).

Individually, or in pairs, create a table top composition in the studio using objects and/or actors. The story evolves from where the objects/actors are placed, the relationship between them (proxemics) and what happens to these relationships over time. Either add a blackout in between the still images or ask the audience to close their eyes while the still image changes and then open them again (Bogart and Landau 149-150).

Excavation Two – walking the grid

Before you start, mark the studio floor into a square with tape. Create a grid of nine equal boxes inside the grid like a tic-tac-toe diagram, or the stage diagram shown in Chapter 5 on No theatre.

Variation: at any point in the explorations, consider redesigning the floor grid to different geometries. What happens when the space is defined as 'lanes' like a swimming pool, or diagonals?

In groups of four, each student chooses one of the Viewpoints and reads the relevant text in Bogart's book. Each student prepares to lead a workshop of 10-15 minutes within their group, teaching them about the chosen Viewpoint: remember the Confucian advice, tell me and I forget, teach me and I may remember, let me teach and I will learn.

Excavation Three – haiku

This exploration comes from Overlie's work with the Six Viewpoints and she simply called it haiku. A haiku is a traditional Japanese poem of three lines of specified number of syllables. Offer both traditional and modern haikus, printed on separate pieces of paper, folded and placed in a hat. For example:

> Between our two lives
> there has lived
> a cherry tree
> (Basho)

> Opening the door –
> oh! oh! oh!
> snow morning
> (Chikamatsu Monzaemon)

> grasshopper –
> do not trample to pieces
> the pearls of bright dew
> (Koboyashi Issa)

> the thief
> left it behind –
> the moon at the window
> (Ryokan Taigu)

Place four shoes in a rectangle to mark a performance space for four performers to move comfortably. In teams of two or four, each performer creates three individual still images to capture each line of their randomly assigned haiku. The still images will be performed inside the arena. The still images are unplanned, but each one must be completely different from each other except that the last still image repeats one element of the first still image but in a different way. Performers enter with their first move, then execute the second move and, finally, the third. Performers shift between their images by sensing the kinesthetic energies of the other performers so that ultimately all move and rest at the same moments. Finish by stepping out of the grid area and standing on the edge at a place of choice, in neutral (Overlie, Haiku Form).

Ask the spectators to comment on the performance. This process causes accidents and coincidences that the spectator will interpret with meaning.

Excavation Four – the walk of life

In pairs, as identical twins, choose a specific character from a book, a play, a film, a TV show. Consider how this character moves in space – with fluid, circular movements; jerky, angular movements; lightly, heavily; weight of feet; point of gravity; and so on. Map the way the character walks on stage as a floor pattern and create a walk of life through the grid as a pair of identical twins.

A topography of your life. Allocate specific meanings to three boxes of the grid. These are moments from your life where significant things happened. Create a still image for each moment. In pairs, as twins, move through and around the grid. When a performer lands on the denoted box of their life, they adopt the relevant pose. Their twin must shadow the still image, before both move on through the grid until all six moments have been shown. Add words, sentences or phrases as desired (Bogart and Landau 56).

Some key concepts from the *Viewpoints* book are included in Table 6.1 if you are looking for extra inspiration. Highlight any boxes you have engaged with and share with a partner.

Table 6.1 Key terms in Viewpoints exploration (Bogart and Landau)

Surrender – you don't have to do it alone; fall back on others, let things happen, don't *make* things happen.	Growth – discover your own strengths and weaknesses. Give yourself time to discover.	'If you can't say it, point to it'.
Soft focus – focus in the distance means you are able to take in more than one thing at a time. Look with the whole body, not just the eyes.	Possibility – there is no right and no wrong, only endless possibilities.	Extraordinary listening – being aware of others in space without needing to look around. Using the body as ears. Get out of your head.
Choice and freedom – endless possibilities mean anything is possible. The more you explore, the more freedom to choose.	Group responsibility – the group is responsible for the physical and mental well-being and safety of all.	Feedforward/feedback Players must give out energy and impulse to initiate as well as when responding.
Change your mind, change what you expect – shift the context to give something a different light, a different way of looking at it.	Don't stay with something until you are finished with it, break off suddenly and do something else.	Fuzzy logic – you can't understand something by studying it too hard, you need to move away from it: the best ideas come when you're not thinking about it.
Actors may share a space in performance but focus on their own material while still aware of what's going on elsewhere. Allow for chance interaction.	Actors are interesting to watch and capable of being watched even though there may not be a role to carry them.	Shift and expand your choreographic frame to everyday activities as you go through your day. Watch the crowd waiting for the train as a performance.

(Continued)

Table 6.1 Continued

Metaphor allows us to look at intense issues without burning our eyes . . . pointing indirectly in order to look at something directly.	Do something unnecessary, not the task in hand. If intending to lift a book, do anything but lift it. How close can you come to doing it, yet stay connected to the task?	Tesseracts: you don't always need transitions. A piece of string can describe a movement from point A to point B. But what happens if you put both ends together? Called a tesseract, it means the spectator can connect in the mind's eye. This is the collaborative work of creation between actor and spectator.
Commitment or, 'wenn schon, dann schon', if you do it, do it. Go all out.	Yes, and . . . is the creative sentence in collaborative devising, followed by Let's try it! There are no buts.	Exquisite pressure – Creating in a compressed amount of time not letting the head get in the way.

In conclusion, whole-class reckoning

Proxemics describe the relationships between objects and bodies in space. Proxemics always generate meaning for the spectator, even if none were intended by the performer.

In order to gain freedom of movement, there are also rules.

Ideas, concepts and aesthetics can travel – between art, dance, music, technology and theatre; between artists, dancers, musicians, designers, actors and computer programmers; and between world theatre forms – from the No stage to the Viewpoints grid.

Resources, Viewpoints

Bogart, Anne. *And then, You Act – Making Art in an Unpredictable World*. New York and London: Routledge, 2007.

Bogart, Anne and Tina Landau. *The Viewpoints Book: A Practical Guide to Viewpoints and Composition*. New York: Theatre Communications Group, 2005.

Buckwalter, Melinda. *Composing While Dancing: An Improviser's Companion*. Madison: University of Wisconsin Press, 2016.

Callery, Dymphna. *Through the Body: A Practical Guide to Physical Theatre*. London: Nick Hern Books, 2001.

Graham, Scott and Steven Hoggett. *The Frantic Assembly Book of Devising Theatre*. London: Routledge, 2014.

Overlie, Mary. "Haiku Form." 2017. Six Viewpoints. 27 January 2020. <https://sixviewpoints.com/haikus>.

—. *The Six Viewpoints*. 2017. 14 February 2020.

Let the people dance a merry jig

The jig is a kind of fast, leaping dance. The name might come from French, giguer – to jump, or Italian, giga – a jump. It was danced solo or in pairs, fours or groups and often accompanied by witty and bawdy lyrics, dramatic inserts, clowning and acrobatics. In Elizabethan and Jacobean theatres, the jig was often 'a conclusion to the theatrical event – whether featured at the close of the drama, or as a dance following the play, or as part of a comic musical afterpiece' (Clegg). Shakespeare's plays often call for a dance or music at the end of the play: music and dance celebrate the four marriages in As You Like It; a march completes King Lear; drums finish off Timon of Athens; and a call for applause completes A Midsummer Night's Dream. The world of play is broken, and the dance, music and song bring the audience back to the real world. Some evidence from earlier Miracle plays points to the idea that the dance at the end of a performance should be enjoyed by actors dancing with the audience, 'Let sum ga drink, and sum ga dance: / Menstrell, blaw vp ane brawl of France; / Let se quha hobblis best' (Let some go drink and some go dance/Minstrel, blow up a brawl in France/Let's see who hobbles the best; Clegg 3). And in 1551, after a performance of Tom Tyler and His Wife, the actor calls, 'Then take hands, and take chance, And I will lead the dance. Come sing after me, and we agree', confirming that spectators were invited to join in the dance with the actors once the play was done (Clegg 3).

The dance at the end of the play not only marked the return to daily life after the fantasy world of play, but its regulated choreography and the beat and rhythm of its music also signified a return to 'safe' world order, where resolution, reconciliation and harmony were restored. At the end of A Midsummer Night's Dream, Bottom asks the Duke if he would like the players to complete their performance of Pyramus and Thisbe with a 'Bergamosque' dance. This was a 'a wanton and rude kinde of musicke' based on the rough and crude manners of the people of Bergamo, possibly influenced by the Commedia dell'arte characters Arlecchino and Brighella, who were natives of Bergamo (Clegg 4). Indeed, it is likely that the character of Bottom was created for Will Kemp, whose personal jig is outlined below. This comic dance by the players, however, is not the end of the actual play, only the play within the play. A Midsummer Night's Dream concludes with Titania and Oberon united, and a 'roundel' of fairies 'hand in hand' in dance and song, restoring the stage world harmony after the chaos of the forest.

Dance is also a great mirror of social hierarchy and divisions:

> It was common for the plots of dramatic jigs to involve the pitting of social types against one another – sometimes divided into those from the country and those from the town – with those of the lowest degree often ending the afterpiece triumphant. Dance was a clear communicator of social type as well as social divisions. (Clegg 11)

The jig at the end of a history play such as Henry IV Part Two 'If my tongue cannot entreat you to acquit me, will you command me to use my legs?' (5.5.17) might re-establish correct social hierarchy. At the end of a romance or comedy, it might re-establish the sanctity of marriage and social conformity as in As You Like It, when the Duke commands, 'Play, music; and you brides and bridegrooms all, /With measure heap'd in joy, to th' measures fall' (5.4.172).

In 1612, the Westminster magistrates decided to 'utterly abolish all jigs, rhymes and dances' at the end of performances, as they were considered rowdy, boisterous and a perfect opportunity for cutpurses to operate, but it seems the tradition did continue, and is continued to this day at the New Globe theatre, as part of their Original Practice mission. Under the direction of Claire van Kampen (Director of Music) and Sian Williams (Master of Dance), the jigs and dances at the end of some plays serve to re-establish and map the character relationships of the play just performed. 'As with all the jigs with which we close plays at the Globe, we celebrate the bond between actors and audience who have journeyed together through the story', says Williams. The jigs at the end of the plays were designed to tell 'complex stories of each character through the choreography' (Clegg 17).

Despite, or because of, its boisterous nature, the jig can return the world to harmony and order again after the chaos and upset of the play world, and it unites the audience and the actors in a lively, happy, activity so that playgoers leave the theatre feeling elevated and cheery. It is with this sense of rambunctious and joyful delight in physical movement, this mapping of circular, unifying topographies, and this coupling and pairing and grouping of everyone engaged in the moment of theatre both actors and spectators, that I invite you to try your hands and feet at this important actor's skill.

Ritual

Around the world, important community moments of everyday life such as the coming of spring, fertility (maypole), summer solstice, love, marriage, harvest, the hunt, overcoming the darkness of winter through fire and light, and chasing the devil with bells and drums are celebrated in music and dance. Many of these dances share simple stepping patterns that repeat over and over again, allowing every participant, of all ages and abilities, to learn the steps/song easily and join in. The dance patterns emphasize open and closed circles – chaining, weaving and promenade walks – and are life-affirming, cyclical, communal activities: everyone moves to the same beat. Many dances are open to any number of participants – traditional line dances, circle dances, as well as weaving dances around a May pole, for example – while others require a partner or groups of partners to make a set. Moving together in rhythm, giving eye contact, hand contact and mixing partners stimulate social interaction, exercise, balance and coordination. The symmetrical and, sometimes intricate, floor patterns made by the dancers are satisfying and pleasing to the eye and the feet. Like the floor patterning of some Asian forms of theatre discussed in this book, the mapping of circles, squares, lines and rows reaffirms the harmony and unity within the community/ ensemble taking part.

Scoring the dance

One of the first pieces of writing on folk dance is by Will Kemp, who was renowned for his comic roles alongside Shakespeare in the theatre company, Lord Chamberlain's Men and likely the actor for whom the role of Bottom in A Midsummer Night's Dream was written (see above). Famed for his jigs, he left the theatre in 1599 and made a 100-mile journey from London to Norwich, dancing jigs all the way to satisfy a bet and raise money. He published a diary of this nine-day tour in 1600, 'Containing the pleasure, pains and kind of entertainment . . . wherein is set down worth note; to reprove the slanders spread of him: many things merry, nothing hurtful. Written by himself to satisfy his friends' (Kemp). Along the way, crowds gathered to watch and sometimes even join in – strangely, twice he recounts young women dancing with him, although women were not supposed to perform in public:

A maid, not passing fourteen . . . made request . . . that she might dance the Morris with me. . . I was soon won; to fit her with bells, besides she would have the old fashion with napkins on her arms, and to our jumps we fell. A whole hour she held out. (Kemp)

Morris dancers used handkerchiefs or pieces of cloth or streamers attached to the shoulders or held between their fingers as decorative elements to emphasize arm movements; sticks and swords for battle/hunting-type dances and bells for chasing evil spirits away and drawing a crowd. In this case, Kemp may have been performing a spring ritual for the growth of the crops since it was said that the higher the Morris dancer leaps, the taller grows the corn (Forbes 62).

A second, important published work is The Dancing Master or Directions for dancing country dances in 1651 (Playford). Here, the author provides over 100 tunes and instructions for dancing to some of them. The names of the dances listed fall into the seasonal categories mentioned above:

Spring: All in a Green Garden, Green Goose Fair, Daphne the Shepherdess, Spring Garden, Green Stockings;
Summer: Sparagus Garden, Rose is white and rose is red, Garland or Summer's day, Dissembling Love or Lost Heart, Chirping of the Nightingale;
Autumn: Catching of quails, gathering of peascods, Jenny Pluck Pears, Jack a Lent, Greenwood or the huntsmen;
Winter: Soldier's Life, Devil's Dream, Drive the Cold Winter Away, Beggar's Boy, An Old Man is a Bed Full of Bones (Playford).

Playford includes descriptions of how to perform the dances and uses the symbol of a round circle with a dot inside for the male dancers (sun) and a dark crescent (moon) for the female dancers, as shown in Figure 6.7. The book describes round dances, longways dances and figure dances for different numbers and, with its sun and moon symbolism for male and female and patterning, links neatly to the topographies of Japanese and Chinese performance spaces, suggesting a universal language of harmonious, symbolic movement linking the performer and the space with nature, the seasons and emotions.

Third, Thomas Bray wrote his Country Dances, being a composition entirely new, in 1699 (Bray), which was published by 'William Pearson next door to the Horse and Feathers'. Both he and Playford describe dancer positions and state that when the female stands on the right of the male it is 'proper' but when she stands on his left, her position is 'improper'. Bray's first entry

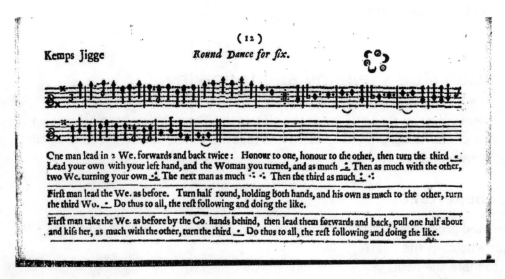

Figure 6.7 Playford's instructions to dance 'Kemp's Jig' 1651 (Playford) © British Library Board, Music Collections K.1.a.12*. Images published with permission of ProQuest. Further reproduction is prohibited without permission.

is a dance called 'The Woman's the Man, A new country dance' and the instruction reads, 'The women begin all improper' (Bray 6). In this dance, the women step to the men in the room and beckon them to dance, and the women take the lead while the men follow. From this, we can see that dance was not just a snapshot celebration of natural or seasonal events, but it could reverse the usual order of masculine and feminine for a moment in time; that it was for simply 'having fun'. It is in this spirit that the following ideas for excavations have been constructed. Instead of masculine and feminine parts in the dance, I suggest the terms *leader* and *follower*.

In this section, online resources provide video examples and tutorials of basic steps and patterns, since it is almost impossible to write down instructions. Moreover, the online sources automatically provide suitable music to start with. But in the end, the best way to learn is to have a go. The dances are taught by doing them, not by reading about them. Encourage the use of the phrase 'can't yet' until students gain proficiency. Let the students know that those who can, should help those who 'can't yet' but who will be able to soon. Ultimately, the movements are designed for everyone and no one should feel left out.

> **Some key vocabulary needed to start:**
> **The closed circle** – everyone faces the centre.
> **Double circle** – one circle inside the other.
> **Lines** – two lines made by pairs.
> **File** – one behind the other in a line.
> **Promenade** – pairs march in file.
> **Chain** – swapping places in the line by handing off left hand, right hand.
> **Set** – groups of couples arranged together.
> **Line of dance** (direction) – always anticlockwise.

Allocate colours for differentiation of leader and follower. If there is an uneven number of participants, one student will become a 'ghost' and execute the dance as if there were a partner present. In this case, choose dance sequences where partners have to change regularly so that everyone gets to dance with a ghost and a partner at some stage. Do not have students 'sitting out'; everyone should join in. It can be helpful to walk through the moves without music first, making sure to count the beats if necessary. The students and the teacher are on the same level of learning – the aim of the session is to share and help each other, not yell instructions and have students standing around waiting for the next step to be explained. Allow students to learn for themselves and from each other.

Excavation One - leading and following

Warm up: music plays as students enter the classroom. There is a written prompt on the board: stand in a circle facing anticlockwise. Feet together. Start with right foot walking forward to a beat. Continue until you stop.

Survey the terrain

What does the group need to make this work?
A caller who calls the beat?
Music to mark the beat?
A cue, 5,6,7,8 or 1,2,3 or ready, and . . .?
A caller who calls the dance to an end?

Excavation Two – closed circle bingo

When teaching partner dance, mark leader and follower roles with coloured bands. This dance requires two distinct groups of dancers that hand off to one another left, and right, in a chain.

Followers and leaders partner up.

Followers create one circle with their leader partners making their own inside circle.

Everyone faces anticlockwise.

Everyone walks to the beat around the circle anticlockwise (see Figure 6.8).

'There was a farmer had a dog,

And Bingo was his name O'

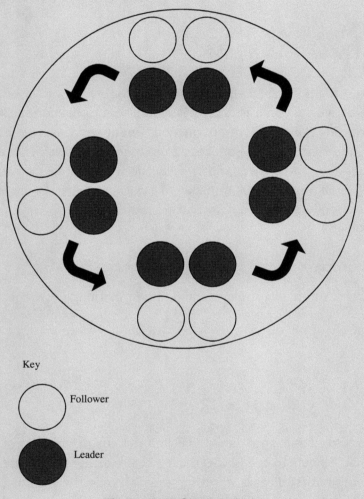

Key

Follower

Leader

Figure 6.8 Closed circle.

Grand right and left: followers step in front of leader partners, facing them, move clockwise and offer first left hand to next oncoming leader dancer, then right hand to following oncoming leader dancer in a weaving pattern passing right shoulders with each other. The leader extends first the left hand to the oncoming follower and then the right to the oncoming follower in a chain around the circle. Keep chaining using alternate left and right hands during the next section of the song:

'B-I-N-G-O

B-I-N-G-O

B-I-N-G-O'

On the final 'O' of this weaving pattern, grand right and left, new partners stop, face each other. Turn anticlockwise again and start the promenade and the song all over again.

'And bingo was his name O'.

Taken from (Pittman, Waller and Dark 66)

Setting the compass

Where does the shoe pinch? What extra tips can students give each other? Are students struggling with left and right? What suggestions do they have for improving this?

Excavation Three – in a line

Saturday Night Fever (Night Fever – Learn to Dance the Steps)

In pairs, browse online for some instructions about how to dance the Brooklyn Shuffle or Saturday Night Fever line dance. There are many different versions; it doesn't matter which you choose. Work out a short-pattern sequence from the video: either forward and back, side to side, hip roll, funky chicken or heel and toe. Pair up with another pair to make a four and combine the moves. Join another four to make an eight and share the moves and so on until the whole class has a sequence of about six patterns.

Roll the music and go!

Resetting the compass

What are the differences between the circle and line formations – how does it feel?

Excavation Four – chaingang

Tanko Buchi is a traditional Japanese dance that imitates the movements of workers in a coal mine digging for coal. Similar to the BINGO dance, it is executed in an anticlockwise circle. The dance has several motifs: digging, throwing the coal over the shoulder, shading the eyes from the moon, pushing the cart, and clapping.

In pairs, students should watch the Tanko Buchi online; there are many examples demonstrating the four different motifs. Learn from watching the dancers.

Once all are comfortable with the motifs, joining the whole class in a circle, moving anticlockwise.

In groups of six, create a chained circle dance similar in style to the Tanko Buchi with four newly invented motifs derived from your own daily life actions. Choose music, share.

Whole-class reckoning

Rhythmical, patterned, repetitive, group movement is an integral part of daily life.

Excavation Five – endless chain

Try the Setnja dance from Serbia. Link arms facing the inside of a circle, but this is a chain, not a closed circle. Anyone can join the line when they're ready.

First, look at the video and practice the steps in pairs.

Starting with right foot, and facing anticlockwise, take two walking steps in the line of direction (anticlockwise circle) to the rhythm of SLOW, SLOW (each step lasts two beats each).

Take two more steps in line of direction QUICK, QUICK.

With right foot, step right and face centre SLOW.

Step left behind right SLOW step right behind left SLOW.

Step backwards left QUICK step right next to left QUICK.

Step left across in front of right SLOW. (Seta)

Think, pair, share

The Setnja increases in speed over time – deliberately forcing mistakes and descending into chaos. Why?

Excavation Six – letting go

Strip the Willow (BBC) – this Scottish dance requires a set of four pairs. Watch the online instruction first, then try it out. Doing is so much easier than watching. Once sets of four have the basics, arrange several sets in the room at one time and watch the willow being stripped!

Think, pair, share

Strip the Willow can get 'boisterous'. Thought-shower in pairs the contrast of control and chaos in dance.

Excavation Seven – the two step

For some calmer action, with a partner, try the two step (Howcast), the two-step promenade (Two Step – The Promenade) and the two step with left turn (Dance).

Once all are comfortable with the step, try a whole-class two step, moving anticlockwise in pairs. Those who are faster should move to the outer edges; the slower dancers keep towards the centre.

Resetting the compass

Distance and proximity, push and pull, lead and follow – are not automatically either masculine or feminine and can shift within a movement sequence.

Excavation Eight - Taminations

Look at the patterning charts in Figure 6.9 (CALLERLAB) and download the app Taminations on the phone. This provides patterns, sequences and dances of all kinds in easy-to-learn animations. Dancers can dance holding the phone as they go!

In sets of six, devise your own dance sequence. Make sure the movements are relevant to daily life actions, nature or include some kind of social purpose such as changing partners.

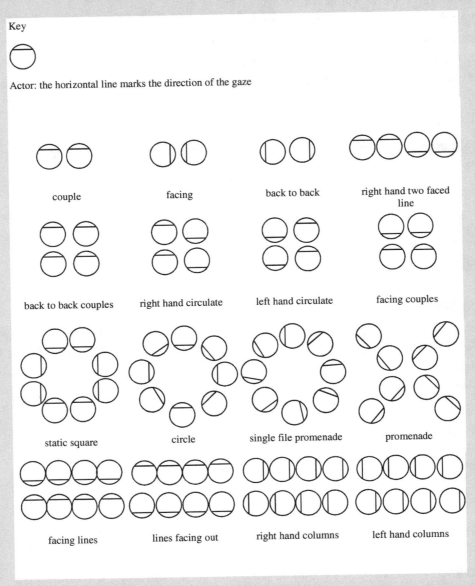

Key

Actor: the horizontal line marks the direction of the gaze

couple   facing   back to back   right hand two faced line

back to back couples   right hand circulate   left hand circulate   facing couples

static square   circle   single file promenade   promenade

facing lines   lines facing out   right hand columns   left hand columns

Figure 6.9 Group movement patterns (CALLERLAB).

Name your dance appropriately and choose music that is the right beat for the moves. It must have:

A circle.
A partner section.
A grand left and right.
An amazing jump.
A dizzying spin.
And two more items of your choice.

And finally: Kemp's jig

To finish this book and return you to the everyday world, although you may not have read this book in sequence, and nor are you required or supposed to do so, here you have landed, at the last pages. So, it seems fitting to offer you the last dance – a jig. This dance is published in Playford's 1651 collection, and though it is named 'Kemp's Jigg' it may not be anything like what Kemp actually danced. But that doesn't matter. It's a sweet, unifying and fun dance to wrap up this gender journey with you.

Round for sets of six people (Norwich Historical Dance)

Start in pairs, standing facing inwards in a closed circle, home positions (see Figure 6.10).

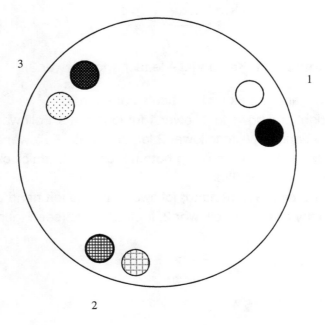

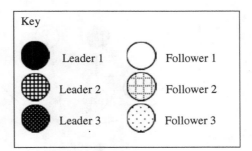

Figure 6.10 Kemp's jig home positions.

All pairs bow to each other.

Leader 1 takes follower 1 by the right hand, follower 2 by the left hand and walks four beats forward towards follower 3, and they all bow to follower 3 for another four beats (see Figure 6.11).

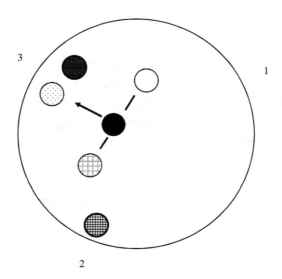

Figure 6.11 Kemp's jig – leader 1 to follower 3.

Leader 1 with followers 1 and 2 walk for four beats backwards.

Leader 1 turns to the right and bows to follower 1 for four beats. Follower 1 returns home.

Leader 1 turns to the left and bows to follower 2 for four beats. Follower 2 returns home.

Leader 1 approaches follower 3 and holding both hands, turns anticlockwise for eight beats before returning follower 3 to home position.

Leader 1 takes follower 3 by the right hand, follower 1 by the left hand and walks four beats forward to follower 2, and they all bow to follower 2, for four beats (see Figure 6.12).

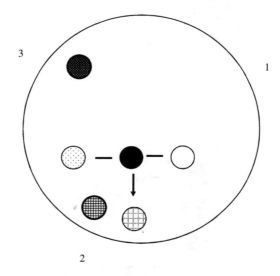

Figure 6.12 Kemp's jig – leader 1 to follower 2.

Leader 1 with followers 3 and 1 walk four beats backwards.

Leader turns to the right and bows to follower 3 for four beats. Follower 3 returns home.

Leader 1 turns to the left and bows to follower 1 for four beats. Follower 1 returns home.

Leader 1 approaches follower 2 and holding both hands, turn anticlockwise for eight beats before returning follower 2 to home position.

Leader 1 takes follower 2 by the right hand, follower 3 by the left hand and walks four beats forward to follower 1, and they all bow to follower 1 for four beats (see Figure 6.13).

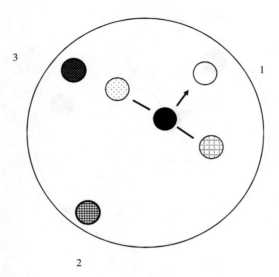

Figure 6.13 Kemp's jig – leader 1 to follower 1.

Leader 1 with followers 2 and 3 walk four beats backwards.

Leader 1 turns to the right and bows to follower 2 for four beats. Follower 2 returns home.

Leader 1 turns to the left and bows to follower 3 for four beats. Follower 3 returns home.

Leader 1 approaches follower 1 and holding both hands, turn anticlockwise for eight beats before returning follower 1 to home position.

Leader 2 takes follower 2 by the right hand, follower 3 by the left hand and walks four beats forward to follower 1, and they all bow to follower 1, for four beats (see Figure 6.14).

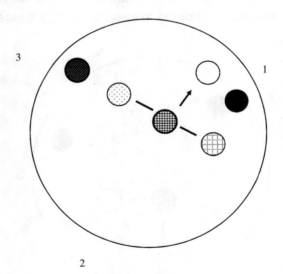

Figure 6.14 Kemp's jig – leader 2 to follower 1.

Leader 2 with followers 2 and 3 walk four beats backwards.

Leader 2 turns to the right and bows to follower 2 for four beats.

Leader 2 turns to the left and bows to follower 3 for four beats.

Leader 2 approaches follower 1 and holding both hands, turn anticlockwise for eight beats before returning follower 1 to home position.

Leader 2 takes follower 1 by the right hand, follower 2 by the left hand and walks four beats forward towards follower 3, and they all bow to follower 3, for four beats (see Figure 6.15).

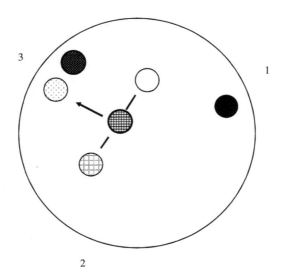

Figure 6.15 Kemp's jig – leader 2 to follower 3.

Leader 2 with followers 1 and 2 walk four beats backwards.

Leader 2 turns to the right and holding both hands, turns anticlockwise with follower 1 for four beats.

Leader 2 turns to the left and holding both hands, turns anticlockwise with follower 2 for four beats.

Leader 2 approaches follower 3 and holding both hands, turns anticlockwise for eight beats before returning follower 3 to home position.

Leader 2 takes follower 3 by the right hand, follower 1 by the left hand and walks four beats forward towards follower 2, and they all bow to follower 2, for four beats (see Figure 6.16).

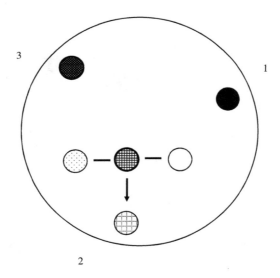

Figure 6.16 Kemp's jig – leader 2 to follower 2.

Leader 2 with followers 3 and 1 walk four beats backwards.

Leader 2 turns to the right and holding both hands, turns anticlockwise with follower 3 for four beats.

Leader 2 turns to the left and holding both hands, turns anticlockwise with follower 1 for four beats.

Leader 2 approaches follower 2 and holding both hands, turns anticlockwise for eight beats before returning follower 2 to home position.

Leader 3 takes follower 3 by the right hand, follower 1 by the left hand and walks four beats forward towards follower 2, and they all bow to follower 2, for four beats (see Figure 6.17).

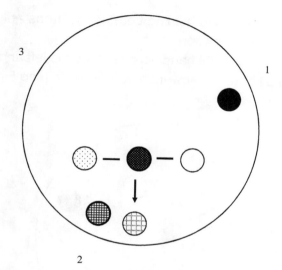

Figure 6.17 Kemp's jig – leader 3 to follower 2.

Leader 3 with followers 3 and 1 walk four beats backwards.

Leader 3 turns to the right and holding both hands, turns anticlockwise with follower 3 for four beats.

Leader 3 turns to the left and holding both hands, turns anticlockwise with follower 1 for four beats.

Leader 3 approaches follower 2 and holding both hands, turns anticlockwise for eight beats before returning follower 2 to home position.

Leader 3 takes follower 2 by the right hand, follower 3 by the left hand and walks four beats forward towards follower 1, and they all bow to follower 1, for four beats (see Figure 6.18).

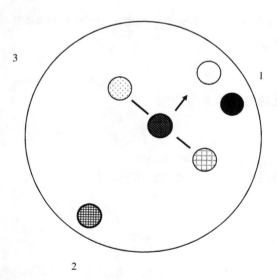

Figure 6.18 Kemp's jig – leader 3 to follower 1.

Leader 3 with followers 2 and 3 walk four beats backwards.

Leader 3 turns to the right and holding both hands, turns anticlockwise with follower 2 for four beats.

Leader 2 turns to the left and holding both hands, turns anticlockwise with follower 3 for four beats.

Leader 2 approaches follower 1 and holding both hands, turns anticlockwise for eight beats before returning follower 1 to home position.

Leader 3 takes follower 1 by the right hand, follower 2 by the left and walks four beats forward towards follower 3, and they all bow to follower 3, for four beats (see Figure 6.19).

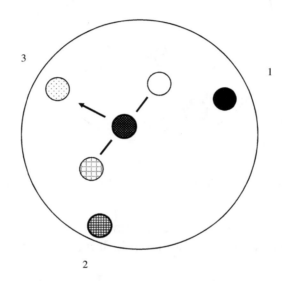

Figure 6.19 Kemp's jig – leader 3 to follower 3.

Leader 3 with followers 1 and 2 walk four beats backwards.

Leader 3 turns to the right and holding both hands, turns anticlockwise with follower 1 for four beats.

Leader 3 turns to the left and holding both hands, turns anticlockwise with follower 2 for four beats.

Leader 3 approaches follower 3 and holding both hands, turns anticlockwise for 8 beats before returning follower 3 to home position.

Everyone has returned home.

In conclusion, whole-class reckoning

The impact of shapes on sense of community.
Movement never ages: tradition versus innovation.
All bodies move in the same way for the same reasons.

Resources, let the people dance

BBC. "Strip the Willow Step-by-Step Guide." 10 December 2013. *BBC One Scottish Country Dancing.* 1 April 2020. <https://www.bbc.co.uk/programmes/p01n4n1l>.
Bray, Thomas. *Country Dances.* William Pearson, 1699.

CALLERLAB Dance Formations, June 2020. <https://www.onemathematicalcat.org/SquareDancing/images/formations.pdf>.

Clegg, Roger. "When the Play is Done, You Shall Have a Jig or Dance of all Treads: Danced Endings on Shakespeare's Stage." *The Oxford Handbook of Shakespeare and Dance*. Oxford: Oxford University Press, 2019.

Dance, Country. "Two Step Dance – The Left Turn." 14 February 2019. *YouTube*. 3 April 2020. <https://youtu.be/RRwV0YBPpsI>.

Forbes, Bronwen. *Make Merry in Step and Song*. Woodbury, MN: Llewellyn Worldwide, 2009.

Howcast. "How to Do the 2-Step." 11 December 2011. *YouTube*. April 2020. <https://youtu.be/xoscqzFdwB0>.

Kemp, Will. *Kemps Nine Daies Wonder. Performed in a Daunce from London to Norwich*. Nicholas Ling, 1600.

"Night Fever – Learn to Dance the Steps." 19 November 2018. *YouTube*. April 2020. <https://youtu.be/ATQmb6UC63A>.

"Norwich Historical Dance." 20 March 2017. *YouTube*. April 2020. <https://youtu.be/GJEj6QsNEf4>.

Pittman, Anne E., Marlys S. Waller and Cathy L. Dark. *Dance A While. A Handbook for Folk, Square, Contra and Social Dance*. San Francisco, CA: Pearson Benjamin Cummings, 2009.

Playford, John. *The Dancing Master, or, Directions for Country Dance*. 1651. Images produced by ProQuest as part of Early English Books Online. www.proquest.com.

Seta. "Seta (Setnja)." 22 December 2012. *YouTube*. 5 March 2020. <https://youtu.be/ATDFVhMWPiU>.

Setnja. "Setnja." 3 November 2008. *YouTube*. March 2020. <https://youtu.be/nxC1e1Q8_Cg>.

"Tanko Buchi." 19 April 2013. *YouTube*. 1 April 2020. <https://youtu.be/Bipj

"Two Step – The Promenade." 4 February 2019. *YouTube*. 3 April 2020. <https://youtu.be/nsk1MPmTrJc>.

INDEX